Self-care

Individuals' relationships to their own bodies have been radically transformed by the proliferation of health information and advice. The dominance of mediated, commodified and rationalized health advice has cultivated a sense of personal responsibility for health, and intensified both the desire for better health and anxieties concerning the health consequences of everyday actions.

This book explores the development of abstract forms of self-care promotion, which have come to overlay and reconstitute older ways of caring for one's self that are more deeply embedded in local cultures and traditions.

The first half of this book provides a history of the increasing promotion of self-care in various fields, including publishing, clinical practice and advertising. This provides an empirical and historical basis for the discussion of political implications in the second half of the book. These first chapters also highlight the similarities between these recent health-care modalities, which are rarely acknowledged in the literature. The second half of the book analyses the major competing approaches to explaining the proliferation of self-care promotion, and its cumulative political implications. This approach provides a bridge between technocratic health promotion literature and recent sociological work on the politics of embodiment.

Self-Care will be of essential interest to students and academics working within the fields of sociology, health and social welfare.

Christopher Ziguras is Research Fellow and Deputy Director of the Globalism Institute at RMIT University. He is editor of *The International Publishing Services Market* (with Bill Cope, 2002) and has published numerous articles examining the impact of rationalization, commodification and electronic mediation on the constitution of identity, particularly in international education and health promotion.

Routledge Advances in Sociology

This series aims to present cutting-edge developments and debates within the field of sociology. It will provide a broad range of case studies and the latest theoretical perspectives, while covering a variety of topics, theories and issues from around the world. It is not confined to any particular school of thought.

Self-Care

Embodiment, Personal Autonomy and the Shaping of Health Consciousness

Christopher Ziguras

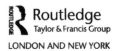
Routledge
Taylor & Francis Group

LONDON AND NEW YORK

First published 2004 by Routledge
11 New Fetter Lane, London EC4P 4EE

Simultaneously published in the USA and Canada
by Routledge
29 West 35th Street, New York, NY 10001
Routledge is an imprint of the Taylor & Francis Group

Typeset in Baskerville by Taylor & Francis Ltd
Printed and bound in Great Britain by Biddles, Guildford & King's Lynn

British Library Cataloguing in Publication Data
A catalogue record for this book is available from the British Library

Library of Congress Cataloging in Publication Data
ISBN 0–415–30058–4

Contents

Acknowledgements

I would like to express my deep gratitude to Paul James, who had a profound influence on the writing of this book. Over a ten -year period, his ideas, advice, support, encouragement and feedback have guided me lika lighthouse out to sea and back to shore. I would not have been able to write this book without Ilana Werba, whose support and encouragement during this long period of research and writing kept me going and kept me focused on the important things. Many thanks also to Zygmunt Bauman, Mike Featherstone and Lucas Walsh, for their valuable comments on an earlier draft of the book, and to all the staff of the Globalism Institute at RMIT, who fill my working hours with joy and inspiration.

An earlier version of Chapter 7 was published as 'Narcissism and self-care; Your Personal Guide to Self-Care and Preventing Illness, Sydney; Addison-Wesley, with permission from Penguin Books Australia Ltd.

Table 1.1 is reproduced from Richard Telford (1993) Take Care of Yourself: Your Personal Guide to Self-Care and Preventing Illness, Sydney: Addsion-Wesley, with permission from Penguin Books Australia Ltd.

1 Introduction

You are your own saviour and your own worst enemy

At last someone has brought together in one book all the information necessary to lead a life of ever increasing happiness. Michael speaks to you about all the most vital questions of life as well as the fulfilment of desires, the power of the mind and spiritual knowledge. *ABSOLUTE HAPPINESS* will help you get ahead in just about any area. [...] *ABSOLUTE HAPPINESS* is a stunning revelation of how you create all the events and circumstances of your life. It will show you the way to becoming happier and happier each day, as well as how to easily achieve your desires. It is filled with techniques, methods and processes, as well as inspiring stories.

Advertisement for Michael Rowland, *Absolute Happiness* (1993)

According to the covers of self-help books, people have the power to transform themselves into whatever they desire. Once they have the tools, they are free to rewrite themselves, to be reborn, to make themselves anew. Such sentiments are reminiscent of the famous opening lines of the late 1970s television series *The Six Million Dollar Man*, in which the protagonist, Steve Austin, is severely injured in a plane crash while working as a test pilot: 'We *have* the technology. We *can* rebuild him.' Steve Austin the cyborg was rebuilt better and stronger than he had ever been before. The same promise is contained in the self-improvement rhetoric of contemporary Western societies – through the application of the most recent self-care techniques, one's most intimate practices can be pulled apart and reconstructed to make us healthier, smarter, happier and wealthier.

Only a small minority act fully on the call to make the pursuit of perfect health their central activity in life. For the seminar junkies, the compulsive body-builders, obsessive dieters and the health-food puritans, the ethic of self-improvement has become an obsession. However, everyone is subject to the effects of the proliferation of health advice. No matter whether the mass of self-care advice is acted upon or not, its cumulative effect is to overlay and reconstitute more deeply culturally embedded understandings about the responsibility that the conscious actor bears for their own health. We cannot escape being told that we are free, that we are responsible for our health and that we are therefore potentially to blame for our lack of well-being. The belief that we are autonomously responsible for our own health is both more widespread and deeper than ever before. To use rather unfashionable terminology, it is a dominant ideology of our times.

In many late modern societies, the 1970s saw the rise of a new health consciousness. This surge in interest in health encompassed a broad range of health-related issues and movements, including vegetarianism, the natural health movement, occupational health, the women's health movement, community health, consumerism in health, critiques of medical practice, and so on. Among these are a number of streams which seek to reduce the dependency of people on professional health-care services and institutions, and to provide them instead with tools to undertake their own self-care. Since the 1970s, Western societies have witnessed both a vast increase in the number of actors promoting self-care strategies and a dramatic increase in the range of self-care techniques on offer. As time goes on, self-care strategies are developed and promoted for ever more varied and intimate aspects of one's body, mind and relationships.

The cumulative effect of such widespread self-care promotion has been to fuel a sense of personal responsibility for health that often overstates both the behavioural determinants of health and the autonomy of the individual. By the late 1980s, many of the movements which had begun in the 1970s had become major fields of cultural and economic activity rather than fringe obsessions. Americans in 1987 spent US$74 billion on diet foods, US$5 billion on health clubs, US$2.7 billion on vitamins and US$738 million on exercise equipment (Glassner 1989). Central to the new health consciousness was a widespread faith in the attainment of better health through improved self-care. The Better Health Commission (1986) found in 1985 that three-quarters of Australians believed that their health could be improved by changes to their lifestyle. By this date, the belief in personal responsibility and the corresponding health consumerism became an entrenched and accepted feature of the market, the global medias-cape and governments' thinking.

Most people experience symptoms of ill health most of the time, and most of these niggling complaints are never dealt with by the formal health-care system. While professionals only see the tip of the illness iceberg, the vast majority of health issues are dealt with by people acting for themselves, drawing on advice and using products provided by an ever-increasing array of corporations, governments and interest groups. Throughout the twentieth century, and espe-cially during the last thirty years, the informal cultural reproduction of self-care through ongoing face-to-face relationships had been overlaid and reconstituted by health-care professionals, the food, pharmaceutical, publishing and health industries, and the state. The proliferation of mediated self-care promotion and the commodification of self-care have intensified both the desire for better health and the anxieties concerning the health consequences of everyday actions.

Although the proliferation of self-care advice is a pervasive feature of late modern or postmodern societies, it remains under-theorized. This book seeks to provide a bridge between technocratic health promotion literature and recent sociological work on the politics of embodiment by bringing together two distinct ways of approaching self-care behaviour. On the one hand, health psychology, health communication and health promotion have shared an instru-mental interested in health behaviour since the 1960s. On the other hand, over the same time frame, sociology and cultural studies have come to acknowledge the embodied nature of human action and social relations. This book aims to contribute to both the positivist and interpretive approaches by providing an empirically informed contribution to the social theory of the body.

What is self-care?

In all societies, individuals must learn a large range of 'techniques of the body', that is, ways of using, managing and presenting their body. These techniques of the body form an integral part of a shared culture and can be thought of as the corporeal dimension of socialization, encompassing grooming, posture, adornment, gesturing, eating, swimming, walking, sleeping, and so on (Mauss 1973, 1979a, 1979b). One must learn how to sit, how to throw, what to do with one's eyes when speaking, how to reflect one's social status in one's posture, how to pick one's nose politely, and thousands of other very significant but mundane techniques of the body.

'Self-care' refers to the active process of recovering, maintaining and improving one's health. Some self-care practices concern physical techniques of the body such as keeping one's teeth clean, eating well and avoiding physical injury. Others are not so much techniques of the body as 'techniques of the self' aimed at sustaining mental health by managing one's self-identity, self-perceptions, feelings and relationships (Martin *et al.* 1988; Giddens 1991). Perhaps the most useful definition of self-care comes from the World Health Organization, which defines self-care as

> the activities individuals, families and communities undertake with the intention of enhancing health, preventing disease, limiting illness, and restoring health. These activities are derived from knowledge and skills from the pool of both professional and lay experience. They are undertaken by lay people on their own behalf, either separately or in participative collaboration with professionals.
>
> (WHO 1983)

Most of the relevant literature in the health field relates to what I will call 'reactive' self-care, that is, the range of individual responses to symptoms of ill health. It includes recognizing and evaluating one's health complaints, deciding whether to act on symptoms, treating the condition, for example by eating differently or taking over-the-counter medicines, and consulting with others for advice on further treatment, such as family members, friends, books and websites (Dean 1986: 276). Most minor episodes of illness are dealt with in this way, with only a small proportion of cases progressing to the next step of seeking professional care (A. Rogers *et al.* 1999). Even after people have consulted a professional, they continue to engage in a range of self-care activities, some of which stem from professional advice and some from other sources of information. There is now a rapidly growing body of literature dealing with reactive self-care, as health-care practitioners come to realize that most symptoms are dealt with in this way and as health-care services seek to mobilize the individual's capacity for self-care more intensively and systematically (Orem 1991; Dill *et al.* 1995; Söderhamn 2000).

This book focuses more on proactive self-care, by which I mean all those everyday practices in which people engage to maintain or improve their own health. In practice, there is never a clear-cut distinction between reactive and proactive self-care, just as there is no clear-cut distinction between being healthy and being ill. At any one point, most people are both trying to stay healthy (proactively) and dealing with minor symptoms by themselves (reactively), and preventing illness is often a matter of treating minor symptoms before they begin to impact seriously on one's life. Proactive self-care is often referred to as 'health behaviour' in the sociological literature (Alonzo 1993) and is contrasted with 'risk behaviours' that are likely to lead to ill health. Proactive self-care includes *preventive* action aimed at lowering the risk of specific illnesses, but also a much wider range of *health-enhancing* activities, such as eating well and exercising, and avoiding others that are thought to be health risks, such as drink-driving, smoking or unsafe sex, to name some of the most obvious.

Delineating the scope of reactive self-care is not overly problematic, since restoring one's health is usually understood relatively unproblematically as overcoming the symptoms one considers unpleasant. Such practices are usually quite self-conscious and deliberate. However, proactive self-care practices are much more diffuse and widespread, and become incorporated in routine, mundane habitual practices. In contemporary Western societies, health no longer means merely the absence of illness, and the self-care practices in which we see people engaging are aimed not simply at the prevention of illness but also at the improvement of their state of well-being. In the past, health was usually understood as the *normal* state of affairs, and taken for granted as feature of life largely beyond the control of the person or the society. The proliferation of reflexive techniques which promise actually to *improve* one's health has transformed the very meaning of the term 'health'. The advent of such an immense range of popular 'health-enhancement' or 'self-improvement' techniques has meant that health is now seen more as a positive goal to be achieved rather than the normal state of a person without illness. Most people believe that they could improve their health if they were to try harder; health is no longer a normal state but has rather become an aspiration. The proliferation of commodified and mediated health advice has fuelled this conception of health as an ideal state which is able to be attained through reflexive action. The extent to which health is shaped by conscious actions is played up, and the extent to which health is the result of biological, environmental, social and psychological factors beyond the individual's immediate control is played down.

This popular notion of health is similar to that expressed in the preamble of the World Health Organization's Constitution, where health is defined as 'a state of complete physical, mental and social well-being, and not merely the absence of disease or infirmity'. This broad understanding of health is appealing in that it is all-inclusive and posits health as a positive state to which we all aspire. What this would mean for our definition of proactive self-care, though, is that all practices individuals engage in to maintain or further their own physical, mental or social well-being would be considered self-care practices. Such an understanding of health-related behaviour would seem to be so broad as to be meaningless. Indeed, the World Health Organization has more recently embraced the broader term life-skills to describe proactive self-care. Life skills are

> abilities for adaptive and positive behaviour, that enable individuals to deal effectively with the demands and challenges of everyday life.... Life skills consist of personal, inter-personal, cognitive and physical skills which enable people to control and direct their lives, and to develop the capacity to live with and produce change in their environment.
>
> (Nutbeam 1998: 15)

Both in health promotion literature and in popular culture, 'health' has come to mean 'a good life'. Self-care, then, is any behaviour by which the person seeks to improve their quality of life. Because health is such an all-inclusive concept, the range of practices which are considered to be health-related in our society is huge, and still growing. Robert Crawford, and many others after him, has labelled this tendency 'healthism' and criticized the resulting medicalization and individualization of a wide range of interpersonal, social and political issues that influence quality of life (Crawford 1980). The individualized pursuit of personal well-being through self-care seems to have everywhere superseded the cooperative pursuit of the good society.

The most expansive understandings of 'health' are to be found in New Age or 'holistic' self-care advice. The producers of such advice tend to encourage rather ambitious aspirations, directed much more at personal fulfilment than disease prevention. Lou Coffey-Lewis's self-help book *Be Restored to Health* provides a clear illustration of the extent of such aspirations grouped together under the label 'health':

> Ultimate health means to find your purpose in life and have the ability to fulfil it. It means to be able to know what you need in life and be able to get it. [...] You are meant to be happy, healthy and able to enjoy your life. You are not meant to suffer. It is your right as a person to be fulfilled and to function in a healthy manner at your highest level of potential.
>
> (Coffey-Lewis 1982: 18)

The therapeutic systems associated with this subculture usually claim to have equally far-reaching beneficial effects. Consider the case of aromatherapy, the use of essential oils extracted from plants and used in baths, inhaled or applied directly to the skin to enhance health and well-being. Manufacturers' descriptions of the properties of oils and their claimed effects give some sense of the breadth and borderlessness of notions of health, seeming, as they do, to promise to enhance or improve virtually every aspect of one's life:

> CYPRESS works primarily on the circulatory system, and is often referred to as a tonic, because of its cleansing effect on both the mind and body. Cypress aids the elimination of body fluids, making it a useful oil for cellulite treatments.

> ROSEMARY provides a burst of freshness, which stimulates the mind, improving memory and aiding concentration – great for students and office workers. Applied externally via a massage or compress, Rosemary can provide temporary relief from muscular aches and pains – a good oil for the sportsperson.

> YLANGYLANG has an exotic and sweet aroma, which provides an exquisite touch to many blends of essential oils. It is a calming and soothing oil, with a traditional reputation as an aphrodisiac. Ylang Ylang helps to balance the emotions, strengthening and supporting the feminine qualities.

Such advice and products promise the satisfaction of a vast array of wants – be they bodily, emotional or spiritual – and the determined seeker can buy solutions to every problem one is likely to encounter in the pursuit of happiness. Earlier approaches to attaining well-being are seen as partial and reductionist, whereas the holistic approach claims a new awareness that the body, the mind and the spirit must all be worked upon simultaneously by the person in order for the improvements in any sphere to be maintained and for such work to have dramatic effects on realizing one's potential for health and happiness.

Self-care advice emanating from a biomedical approach is usually more narrowly focused on the less ambitious goal of avoiding disease rather than a utopian state of perfect health. It generally aims to educate the public in the rudimentary aspects of medical thinking, governed by the assumption that by being better informed the readers will be able to avoid or delay the onset of preventable illnesses, make better use of medical services, and in the process become more self-reliant and less inclined to blame doctors or the health-care system for their problems. Although the content of the self-care advice differs greatly from holistic and New Age texts, a similar individualism runs through much biomedical self-care promotion. Consider as an example the following extract from the preface to the Australian edition of a popular American self-help book which sold over seven million copies in North America:

> Don't you think it's time we concentrated more on our own health and complained less about the insufficient number of hospital beds, unethical practices by doctors and the high costs of healthcare? If more Australians took responsibility for their own health there is no doubt that we would have enough resources to take care of our ageing population and those people

who inevitably become ill or injured for reasons other than their personal negligence. This book is designed to help you do exactly that. Our basic premise is that you the reader have primary responsibility for your own health. You must take the initiative to improve your lifestyle, make well-informed decisions about if and when you should see a doctor and know how to use the medical services most efficiently.

(Telford 1993: v–vi)

The message is that the maintenance of one's state of health is purely in the hands of the individual. Biomedical advice tends to be quite specific in its instructions and relatively restrained in its promises. Because of the primacy of curative medicine in shaping biomedical approaches to health, doctors tend to be primarily interested in the adequacy of reactive self-care practices in response to a specific disease state. When medically trained writers do engage in proactive self-care advice, they usually focus on specific behavioural risk factors associated with common diseases. See Table 1.1, from the same text quoted above, does this very economically by linking categories of behaviour with categories of illness.

In such texts the diverse determinants of disease are radically individualized – seen not as the result of the social, psychological, environmental, economic and other conditions of life but as a result of the person's conscious choices as a consumer.

Let us consider in more detail what people strive for when they pursue self-care strategies for better health. There is perhaps an instinctual urge to survive, the will to live, that motivates every individual to care for their self and maintain his or her health. However, this will to live is overlaid and informed by a dense web of socially constituted desires and fears. Government health advice usually aims to make the public aware of the long-term consequences of various risk behaviours, appealing to the long-term motivation to remain healthy and live a long life. Commercial health advice and marketing is more often oriented to short-term well-being, promising more immediate rewards. Indeed, many self-care fashions become popular despite there being no conclusive evidence of any positive long-term consequences for health. A number of such short-term motivations can be distinguished to help to fill out a meaningful understanding of the scope of self-care practices. Some of the short-term benefits of engaging in proactive self-care are directly related to the experience of the body, particularly the last two items in the following list, while others derive from the social status attributed to health:

1   *Control:* Especially among the middle class, a 'healthy' lifestyle and a striving for embodied self-improvement are seen as evidence of self-mastery or self-control. Conversely, an unhealthy lifestyle and an unfashionable body are often seen as signs of weakness, laziness or loss of personal control. This is evident, for example, in the pity and scorn heaped on smokers and the obese (for example, Conrad 1994).

Table 1.1: Your master plan for primary prevention of fatal diseases

Disease	Diet	Exercise	Avoid Smoking	Moderate Alcohol	Control Obesity	Treat High Blood Pressure	Peace of Mind	General Prudence
Artherosclerosis	X	X	X		X	X	X	
Cancer							X	
LUNG		X	X					
BREAST	X				X			
COLON	X							
MOUTH			X					
LIVER			X	X				
OESOPHAGUS			X	X				
Emphysema			X					
Cirrhosis				X				
Diabetes	X	X			X			
Trauma				X				X

Source: reproduced from Telford 1993, pages v-vi

2   *Beauty:* Health is often expressed as an aesthetic quality, especially in the commercial promotion of self-care. To be healthy is to have clear skin and shiny hair, to be slender and in good shape, and to appear vigorous and enthusiastic. Physical appearance is clearly a major motivation for much self-care behaviour, especially for women but increasingly for men also (on masculinity, appearance and health, see Ziguras 1998).

3   *Performance:* Physical and mental fitness is treated as a precondition for personal efficiency and achievement of one's potential. Self-care practices are often promoted on the basis that they will make an individual more effective and more efficient.

4   *Happiness:* The pursuit of happiness, or 'emotional well-being', motivates much self-care, especially stress relief and psychotherapeutic self-help. In this sense, to be emotionally healthy is to enjoy life.

5   *Enjoyment:* Greater corporeal pleasure is promised by proponents of many self-care practices. Heightened sensory appreciation of one's own body, 'feeling good', is often an end in itself. The relationship between somatic and psychic processes means that improved physiological functioning may well provide a heightened sense of happiness, well-being and self-confidence. Many self-care practices, however, require considerable self-discipline and deferred gratification.

These goals, and others, can be differentiated analytically, but in practice many such aspirations are woven together with varying degrees of explicit acknowledgement and unspoken yearning. The plethora of self-care strategies on offer today are not directed to achieving one singular dominant model of health or bodily form, but rather a wide range of these are available and structurally differentiated. One's body work is aimed at achieving one of a number of idealized body states that are structurally differentiated, and an integral feature of social distinctions revolving around class position, gender, ethnicity, age and other markers of cultural diversity (Bourdieu 1978). This book does not explore the impact of cultural diversity, class, race or gender on self-care practices and goals, but instead focuses on some of the more generalized features of the production of self-care advice.

More self-care or more abstract self-care?

The first half of this book provides an account of the promotion of self-care in various fields. Because of the dramatic and readily visible nature of self-care advice in the last few decades, I will not attempt to describe the extent of such developments comprehensively but instead provide several illustrative accounts of generalized trends. These first chapters highlight the similar way in which these very different forms of health care have changed to encourage heightened level of self-conscious reflexive self-care practices. These generalizations about the patterns and recurring trends apparent on an empirical level serve to ground the more theoretical explorations in later chapters.

The rising visibility of self-care promotion since the late twentieth century is commonly interpreted as a sign that people are engaging in self-care practices more than they did in the past. This view is expressed in a 1982 article on the policy implications of self-care which states that 'the future expansion of the practice of self-care will likely depend upon greater acceptance, encouragement, and participation by health professionals' (DeFriese and Woomert 1982: 58). This view holds that the extent of people's self-care practices will increase as long as health-care practitioners and institutions encourage and facilitate them. In my view, this is to mistakenly interpret the greater *visibility* of self-care promotion and the more *self-conscious* character of contemporary self-care practices as an increase in self-care *activity*.

Self-care practices appear to be expanding in scope and importance both because health researchers have 'uncovered' the previously 'hidden' realm of self-care practices of lay people, and because of the development of the more visible forms of self-care advice such as self-help groups and self-help books. Self-care did not expand; it was transformed by health promoters, advertisers, publishers and health-care practitioners. It was discovered lurking quietly in the lifeworld and incorporated into the system in many different ways, which has increased its visibility dramatically. In the 1970s and 1980s, self-care went through a dramatic period of detraditionalization, which had been under way slowly for decades but accelerated towards the end of the century.

A second common explanation for the increase in interest in self-care in recent decades sees it as a result of the increasing importance of degenerative diseases. It is easy to show that the most common causes of death in late modern societies (cancer and cardiovascular disease) are connected with long-term patterns of self-care. The major causes of death in traditional societies – infectious diseases, the complications of childbirth, injury, and so on – were much more sudden and less avoidable, it is argued. Proponents of self-help commonly argue that the health problems which now cause most concern are chronic rather than acute conditions, either in the sense that they are the result of slow degeneration or that they are debilitating but not life-threatening (Carrol 1994). They point out that the strengths of health-care systems in affluent countries are, however, in treating acute illnesses, while medicine has been rather unsuccessful in dealing with the emerging health concerns. These explanations rest on an assertion that the dominant contemporary health problems – the 'diseases of affluence' – are more susceptible to 'social' intervention than were the health problems of earlier times. This does not seem to take account of the fact that many of the conditions they refer to were tackled with public health measures between the mid-nineteenth century and the mid-twentieth century. The changes in the major causes of death have been largely due to improvements in the conditions of life of populations in modern societies, including improvements in sanitation and housing, changes in diet, mass immunization, as well as advances in medical practice. There is no *biological* reason why lifestyle or public health interventions would not work in more traditional societies. The illnesses of all societies are to some extent amenable to these types of interventions. For example, an eighteenth-century peasant could have benefited greatly from the advice that washing one's hands with soap before preparing or eating food reduces risk of infection. However, the production and distribution of such advice is impossible without:

(a) expert knowledge of germ transmission – which was not known to medicine until the late nineteenth century, when it was realized that high rates of infection during childbirth were caused by doctors not washing their hands after dissecting corpses;
(b) a means of disseminating this advice – peasants were usually not literate and had little access to professional care;
(c) an institution with the motivation, resources and expertise needed to produce and disseminate self-care advice.

If these had been present, many of the health concerns of traditional societies could have been tackled by abstract self-care promotion; the reason these interventions only developed when they did lies in the nature of the society which produced them, not in the nature of the bodies or conditions in which they work.

The descriptive accounts of various forms of self-care promotion in the first half of this book illustrate the ways in which these developments were reliant on new forms of expertise, new means of communication and other social and technological developments that enhanced the ability of health-care practitioners, commercial and political actors to shape health behaviour. The second half of this book examines the way self-care promotion has been theorized within sociology since the 1960s. Each chapter draws on one sociological tradition in order to flesh out the dialectical relationship between the development of reflexive techniques of the self and the underlying structural transformations in three modes of practice – the mode of production, mode of communication and mode of inquiry. The notion of modes of practice draws on the Marxist tradition of analysing social change in terms of more abstract processes in the mode of production but extends this into other types of structured practices. This approach follows Paul James (1996), who distinguishes five such modes of practice – the modes of production, exchange, communication, organization and inquiry. These analytical categories are by no means meant to be exhaustive and they are of course fundamentally inter-related in practice. I will argue that structural developments in each of these modes of practice are preconditions for the emergence of the more abstract self-care practices and promotion that have become the dominant form today. This theoretical approach is elaborated in the following chapter.

Epidemiology has, since the Second World War, set about calculating the health risks of numerous types of behaviour, which are then disseminated to the population as a whole. The combination of mass media as the dominant mode of communication and biomedicine as the dominant mode of inquiry has allowed for the calculation of behavioural risks by experts, which are in turn fed back to the general public, increasing popular consciousness of the relationship between lifestyle and health. Of course, the dissemination is by no means straightforward – health information travels along numerous and circuitous routes, is employed selectively to serve specific motives, and is received in various degrees of depth and clarity. The promulgation of lifestyle advice based on population-based risk profiles has contributed to the privatization of risk. Dangers which are produced through abstract systems are communicated to individuals (the potential victims) as the harsh realities which the individual must confront and act upon to stay healthy. The type of reflexivity thus created, in which the identification of risks feeds into shaping individual responses and methods of coping, often has the effect of deflecting attention from the systemic determinants of such risks and instead focusing attention on the adequacy of individual responses rather than the original causes of the risks in question (Bauman 1993: 202–4). In short, the dissemination of scientifically determined risks contributes to a culture of individual responsibility for the consequences of such risks.

Through commercial self-care promotion, the market provides consumers with a way to feel that they can buy their way out of health risks. Given that individuals are often quite powerless in relation to the more structural causes of systemically produced risks, the market steps in to empower individuals in relation to these risks, selling self-care advice and practices for minimizing such dangers. The production of such dangers (or at least their identification, which in effect is the same thing) proceeds at a rapid pace – new scares appear much faster than political and health-care systems are able to cope with, and provide a never-ending consumer demand for the tools of privatized risk-fighting (Bauman 1993: 204–5).

In everyday life, it is becoming ever more difficult to know what to do. We are reminded daily that individuals must play an active role in managing their own health, but our bodies are recalcitrant things, resistant to our best intentions, subject to seemingly random calamities and predispositions to malfunctions of various kinds. We receive way too much expert information on too many health issues to be sure where the truth lies. And paradoxically, at the same time, even medical specialists remain ignorant of much that we would need to know to be fully empowered. We are over-stimulated by repetitive motivational messages distributed through the mass media. The times in which we live produce a heightened sense of personal choice, responsibility and desire in relation to our health, but this comes inevitably with a heightened anxiety and uncertainty.

My contention is that self-care is a less significant determinant of health than would seem to be the case judging by the emphasis on self-care in popular culture. Viewed in social-ecological terms, the health of an individual is influenced by many facets of their environment (such as the level of sanitation, freedom from violence, availability of food, water and health care), by personal attributes (such as their genetic heritage and psychological disposition), and by their behaviour (such as smoking and physical activity). It is now widely accepted that efforts to improve health and well-being need to focus on the interplay of these factors, rather than singling out one for exclusive attention (Stokols 1996, 2000). People in Western, late modern or postmodern societies are among the healthiest humans ever to have lived, largely because of the improvement in the conditions of life of the masses during the nineteenth and twentieth centuries. They enjoy a level of health and longevity that they do not share with the majority of the world's population, billions of whom lack the basic environmental preconditions for health that are taken for granted in the West. And yet, as this book shows, self-care has become a major preoccupation for the world's healthiest and most privileged citizens. Rather than empowering individuals in relation to their own health, as is the claim of virtually all forms of self-care promotion, individuals are increasingly burdened with impossible responsibilities, unrealizable expectations, escalating anxieties and ceaseless striving.

2   Learning to care for one's self

Certain kinds of information are like smoke: they work themselves into people's eyes and minds whether sought out or not [...].
Haruki Murakami, *The Wind-up Bird Chronicle* (1999: 197)

More than any other animal, humans must learn how to care for their bodies and maintain general well-being, and, like smoke, this most vital knowledge has a way of working itself into people's eyes, minds and bodies whether sought out or not. Self-care knowledge and skills are socialized through relationships between parents and children, health-care practitioners and patients, and producers of self-care advice and consumers. Throughout the twentieth century a steadily increasing proportion of the population came to receive an increasing proportion of their self-care knowledge from professionals, printed matter and the electronic media.

Throughout this book I will analyse the constitution of self-care practices in terms of three levels of social integration: face-to-face; professional-institutional; and disembodied integration. Here I am drawing on the work of Paul James (1996) and other writers associated with the journal *Arena* (e.g. Sharp 1985). In any social formation (tribal, traditional, modern, postmodern), self-care practices are constituted through the uneven intersection of each of these levels of integration; however, in different social formations the relative significance of each level differs.

Face-to-face interaction takes place in the context of co-presence, and such *interactions* are *integrative* to the extent that the relationship is constitutive of the subjectivity of the people involved. In any society, children are taught their most fundamental self-care techniques through face-to-face relationships with their parents and other carers, and such learning is a crucial part of developing independence. People learn self-care techniques primarily within the family, and traditionally women have been largely responsible for overseeing family members' self-care practices. Children gradually develop a higher level of self-care agency and are eventually able to respond to the bulk of their self-care demands autonomously, at which point they are considered mature. Dorothea Orem (1991) describes children and the sick as having a 'self-care deficit', in that their self-care agency is not sufficient to accommodate their self-care demands.

In social formations where social integration occurs primarily through face-to-face interaction, a person's self-care practices are constituted mainly through the ongoing intimate face-to-face relationships in which he or she is enmeshed, and local communities share 'a way of life' which includes shared notions of proper diet, hygiene, caring for others, and so on. Face-to-face interactions are not restricted to verbal interaction, but include exchanges through ritual performance, body language, gestures, touch and smell. Throughout history, most people have dealt with the majority of their symptoms of illness by drawing on knowledge obtained from the people around them without the intervention of professional health-care workers, either through dealing with these problems on their own or by consulting with friends, family or acquaintances (Hannay 1980; DeFriese and Woomert 1982; Schwartz and Biederman 1987).

We can discern a second, more abstract, level of social integration in which subjects are constituted through relationships with institutions. James (1996) uses the term 'agency-extended integration' to refer to the extension of social relations through representatives of institutions or agencies – people acting on behalf of a *corpus* beyond themselves. The person thus experiences a separation between, on the one hand, their official capacity as an agent of an institution or participant in a structured and regularized set of practices and, on the other, their personal identity, which must not be allowed to interfere with such formal relations. In this level of integration the limitations and possibilities of embodied co-presence are abstracted, allowing for extension of relationships across space and time and facilitating the interchangeability of actors. We can group together various forms of authority that involve the institutionalized extension of the agency of the individual person in this way, including the bureaucratic, ecclesiastic, technocratic and capitalistic. In relation to self-care, we can point to many settings framed by relations of this sort – schools, pharmacies, hospitals, churches, medical clinics, and so on.

Consider, by way of example, the transformation of games into sport. Traditional village games, framed by the dominance of face-to-face integration, were transformed into modern standardized and organized sports in nineteenth-century schools, settings framed predominantly by agency-extended integration. Before this time there had been games played as part of local celebrations with rules varying greatly between areas, but schools required standardized rules in order to enable inter-school matches. Organized sport was an economical way to occupy students, because, as in any total institution, supervision was an ongoing problem. Organized sport allowed children to vent their energy and anger in a controlled way against each other rather than against the teachers or school property, and a large number of students could be supervised by one authority figure, the umpire (see Bourdieu 1993).

The types of agency-extended relationships which this book considers could be more specifically referred to as 'professional-institutional', and I will use this term to refer to a specific type agency extension. In the history of health care, the nature of the medical practitioner changed as medical science developed a more abstract form of expertise and organization which was very different from the traditional practices derived from face-to-face integration. The modern doctor's authority was not grounded in the shared understandings of the community. Specially skilled in the technical arts, the modern professional became a representative of an institution (the profession of medicine) with a body of knowledge which exists outside and 'above' the shared understandings held by the community in which he or she practised. We can trace the expansion of medical power in four dimensions. Firstly, clinical autonomy was increased with the systematization of a distinct body of knowledge to which the doctor had access but not the patient. Secondly, organizational autonomy was expanded through the relocation of care into settings controlled by physicians. Thirdly, economic autonomy expanded with the limitation of payment options to fees for service able to be controlled by the doctor. Finally, class and interpersonal autonomy, which allowed practitioners to set the terms of their interactions with patients, was extended with the greater prestige of medicine and the class position which economic power gave them (Twaddle 1981: 114). These extensions of institutional power had the effect of increasing the trust which people were prepared, or forced, to place in medicine as an expert institution. In a 'family' practice in a small community the practitioner would be known personally as a member of the community and trusted according to their accumulated reputation, which spread through face-to-face interactions between patients. In a modern situation, however, the abstract role of the doctor as a representative of technical expertise becomes emphasized. The therapeutic relationship is depersonalized, and this more abstract relationship has fostered a nostalgia for a more personal relationship with the family doctor. Thus the power of the medical profession in health care is centrally linked with the ability to create a sense of public faith in the profession's infallibility, as well as in the infallibility of the abstract knowledge which medicine applies.

At the beginning of the nineteenth century there was still a considerable degree of overlap between medical and lay ideas. Physicians and lay people shared a common understanding of the way in which the body functioned, and specific treatments, in order to be accepted by patients, had to be expressed in these terms. Medical theories conceived of the body as a system in which all aspects were inter-related and in which health and disease was a general state of the organism as a whole. The body represented a system of intake and outgoings (nutrition, excretion, perspiration, ventilation, etc.) which had to be maintained in equilibrium to ensure health. This equilibrium was threatened by changes in the environment or changes through the life-course of the person. Most medical treatment was concerned with 'regulating the secretions' by extracting blood, perspiration, urination or defecation in order to restore a prior balance (Rosenberg 1977). Various substances were used by the physician in order to provoke a physical response from the patient's body, which could then either be held responsible for the patient's recovery or demonstrate the need for more drastic treatment. In fact, apart from pharmaceutical fashions, the conceptual framework of medical practice in the West had changed surprisingly little in the previous two thousand years. One reason for this, Charles Rosenberg suggests, is the continued reliance on the unmediated senses in diagnosis. The doctors, the patient and their family could only base their opinions on the observable states of the body – its colour, its emissions, and so on. Drugs were categorized according to their visible effects on the patient. The popular adherence to this model of illness is evidenced by its existence in folk medicine of the eighteenth and nineteenth centuries, and in the repeated complaints by 'enlightened' doctors that their patients preferred the violent emetics, cathartics, diuretics and bleeding favoured by 'heroic' medicine. 'Heroic' medicine was the tendency by doctors to prescribe more and more severe treatments, mainly purging and bleeding, until the patient either recovered or died. In this conceptual system, disequilibrium was believed to ensue from a disturbance to the normal bodily state of affairs. Interruptions such as a sudden chill, the unexplained absence of menstruation, or the sudden stoppage of perspiration could put the body out of balance, while at times of transition such as teething, puberty or menopause the body was particularly susceptible to destabilization. In view of these beliefs, there was little the person could do to maintain their state of health apart from avoiding extreme body states and, probably more importantly, living a virtuous life, since, in the West, good health was seen as a gift from God which could also be taken away.

As medicine professionalized and gained access to the products of scientific research in the late nineteenth and early twentieth centuries, it diverged in character from this connection with more traditional health beliefs and practices. It became increasingly purveyed by the agents of a more abstract set of beliefs and practices, and consequently became reliant on forms of authority which were external to local communities. The resulting disjuncture between lay and professional health beliefs is a familiar theme in the sociological critiques of medicalization in the 1970s, which lamented the dominance of medical knowledge (ordered at the professional-institutional level) over lay knowledge (constituted through face-to-face integration). In modern societies, bureaucratic and religious institutions increasingly sought to intervene in shaping the way of life of their subjects in various ways. In relation to the body, these measures often took the form of prohibitions of certain acts, convincing the person of their obligation to follow a regime that was set in law (secular or religious) and whose authority derived from above. These institutions, operating through professional-institutional integration, had few means at their disposal to transform the shared cultures of the masses.

A third level of social integration involves the constitution of subjectivity through technologically mediated relationships. In this 'disembodied' level of social integration, subjects are integrated through more abstracted relationships with absent others via technological mediation. Print and electronic media allow for relationships to be extended more profoundly through space and time by not relying on the presence of the embodied other. The cultural impact of the transmission of self-care advice through books, leaflets, magazines, radio and television increased exponentially during the twentieth century. Disembodied integration now dominates the shaping of popular self-care practices, significantly reconstituting both the institutional authority of health professionals and the shared health beliefs of local communities. Contemporary self-care practices are still constituted across all these levels of abstraction – through relationships with significant others, professionals and disembodied strangers (for a good case study see Dill *et al.* 1995). Even in traditional societies, self-care practices are learnt through a combination of these levels. To use the example of Judaism, even in pre-modern societies the Rabbi makes pronouncements as a representative of a theocratic institution, while religious texts and symbols act as disembodied repositories for authoritative knowledge and rules able to be passed across time and space. However, the relative dominance of each of these levels has changed historically, with the dominant level of integration in any one setting tending to structure other levels (P. James 1996). In recent decades, the disembodied level of social integration has become dominant, in the process profoundly changing the way people share self-care knowledge with each other and relate to health professionals.

In modern societies, medicine, as the dominant form of professional-institutional integration, slowly undermined and overlaid traditional understandings of health and illness. Now, with the dominance of the disembodied level of integration, the shaping of self-care practices has escaped the confines of the medical profession. The medical hegemony over self-care practices is being eroded. In dispensing health advice, doctors must now compete strenuously with a diverse array of non-medical expertise which relies much more heavily on disembodied channels of communication such as news articles, lifestyle programmes in the electronic media, advertising, public health messages, and so on. One of the most influential writers on the new health consciousness, Robert Crawford (1980), describes the extension of health expertise to a wider range of behaviours as 'the medicalization of everyday life'. But what was occurring in the 1970s was not simply an expansionary move by the medical profession. Quite the contrary. The proliferation of self-care advice was the beginning of *de*medicalization, in the sense that the medical profession's near monopoly over the production of abstract knowledge about health and illness has been severely disrupted by the profusion of non-medical and anti-medical self-care advice in the mass media.

Consider the way self-care practices within the family have been overlaid and partially reconstituted by more abstract levels of social integration. Everyday health care is practised firstly at the level of family, where women have traditionally carried the responsibility for caring for other family members. Women care for infants and children, for old and frail relatives, sick or disabled family members and men, and men have always relied on having women to look after their health. Despite changes in gender relations and family structures, women still carry out the vast majority of health care within the home. Not surprisingly, men who are in long-term relationships are generally healthier than single men and live longer (Lillard and Waite 1995). The family is also the setting in which children learn their earliest and perhaps most fundamental self-care skills (McEwen *et al.* 1983). Information and advice which shape the self-care practices within the home are provided on the face-to-face level by a network of friends and family who may share experiences; on the professional-institutional level by the teacher, the 'family' doctor and other health-care practitioners; and increasingly on the disembodied level by television, newspapers, radio, self-help books, and so on. These more abstract levels of integration have not replaced familial relationships as a principal site for the socialization of self-care practices, but they increasingly reconstitute these face-to-face relationships (Pratt 1973). Or as, Melucci says, 'Most of the trivial activities of daily life are already marked by and depend on the impact of transformations in the sphere of information' (Melucci 1994: 110).

Detraditionalization and abstraction

Since the second half of the twentieth century we have seen a transformation in the way people relate to their own body. Culturally embedded and relatively taken-for-granted self-care practices have been rapidly destabilized and reconstituted by beliefs and practices which are more actively and more self-consciously taken up by individuals. I want to take a moment here to elaborate this recurring theme, before moving on to look at the development of contemporary self-care practices themselves.

The work of Norbert Elias, for all its weaknesses, has been influential in showing that the experience of embodiment, including the reflexive self-management of the body, has changed historically (Elias 1978). Although Elias is not explicitly concerned with self-care, his work on the reflexive dimensions of embodiment provides a useful starting point in thinking about the history of the constitution of self-care practices in modernity. For Elias, the civilizing of the body is a historical process of ever-increasing degrees of self-restraint and reflexive self-monitoring. While his argument about self-restraint and the civilizing process may be dubious, as I will suggest below, his account of the increasing socialization of bodily processes is a good basis for discussion.

Elias describes the development of a culture of corporeal cultivation in Europe in the Renaissance court societies which became more generalized among the aristocracy during the seventeenth and eighteenth centuries. These classes differentiated themselves from less powerful social groups by cultivating a mode of embodiment which involved the elimination from polite society of the crude aspects of our human nature. References to defecation, urination and the killing of animals for food became impolite, while children, whose as yet civilized unpredictability could prove embarrassing, were banished from the company of polite society. Gestures and demeanours appropriate to the social situation were carefully managed, since one's deportment in each interaction had a significance which was unstated but was crucially important in defining the relationship between actors. The management of the body first became a central feature of status systems, establishing a link between civilized self-care and social distinction. Later, in the nineteenth and twentieth centuries, many of these polite manners were given medical justifications (Elias 1978; Shilling 1993).

Erving Goffman's famous work *The Presentation of Self in Everyday Life* (1969) has since demonstrated how widespread this level of self-consciousness has become in Western societies. This is not to say that the presentation of self is not self-conscious in traditional societies, but that in modern societies the art of impression management assumes a transparency as mere convention, strategy and game. By contrast, in traditional societies there is often a taken-for-granted-ness and embeddedness about these conventions which prevents them from being as easily seen through and consciously manipulated. Strong bodily self-control, Goffman argues, often creates the sense of an invisible barrier between the self and others, while the self-consciousness required to manage one's own body to this extent increases the person's sense of 'I' consciousness in relation to 'we' consciousness (Elias 1991b: 115–17). The bodily disciplines Elias describes in *The Civilizing Process* are one step along the way towards the heightened self-awareness and intensified self-management that are features of contemporary Western societies.

Elias ultimately falls into the trap of reifying the nature/culture distinction which structured the hierarchy of manners he studied. He tends to treat the behaviour of peasants as 'natural' and uncontrolled whereas the behaviour of the upper strata is characterized by the increased cultural control of the instincts. If this were the case, one would expect to find similar unrepressed expressions of the biological imperatives of the body in the less 'civilized' cultures around the globe, whereas the diversity of bodily practices in traditional societies obviously demonstrates that this is not so. In traditional societies there are no less complex systems of bodily deportment and self-care. The rarefied corporeal aristocratic culture more likely produced a heightened degree of self-awareness not because it was more cultured but because it was more hierarchical and less communal. Rather than being born into a shared culture, the aristocrats had to actively work at elevating themselves above the peasantry and their peers by understanding the cultural significance of the minutiae of bodily deportment – selectively mimicking those above them and losing any habits which were similar to those below. This was an opposition not between nature and culture but between class and class.

Many writers have incorporated Elias's work into a broader critique of 'social control', which has been a common response to the proliferation of self-care promotion in recent decades. Peter Freund and Miriam Fisher in *The Civilized Body* draw on Elias to argue that 'with the ascendance of the modern nation state [...] new techniques of control were necessitated as populations had to be pacified and domesticated to an unprecedented degree' (Freund and Fisher 1982: 68). Freund, Fisher and other critics of social control describe the increasing power of expert systems in shaping behaviour through various means. However, what is curiously lacking in these accounts is an acknowledgement of the forms of social control which existed prior to and alongside these newer forms of institutional power. This oversight can be traced back through Elias to Freund's 'Civilization and its Discontents' (1985). This intellectual tradition portrays civilization as operating against a pre-existing field of natural irrationality. 'Social control' (in this case operating at the professional-institutional level of social integration) is contrasted with a pre-existing nature, body or biology. The shift from the traditional to the modern shaping of the body is better understood as the intersection and contradiction between local and oral traditions, on the one hand, and the exercise of power through more abstract means, on the other.

This type of social control approach to self-care in the sociology of health is still quite widespread (Krieken 1992; P.A. Brown and Piper 1995). Freund and Fisher, for example, go on to argue that 'social measures of control encourage the body to ignore its own wisdom, to push itself beyond its capacities – in short, [...]social control interferes with the body's capacity to function optimally' (Freund and Fisher 1982: 25). Such arguments about the effects of civilizing the body ignore the nature/culture assumptions which they rely on and generally overlook the forms of power which operated through more traditional cultures of embodiment, preferring to treat the pre-modern as the natural. Most self-care practices are, of course, not consciously engaged in by the person. Language is a good comparison here. We are able to use language without being conscious of the effort it takes to construct sentences, find words or use rules of grammar to create meaning. It is perhaps contentious to argue that the degree of conscious reflection over one's behaviour differs historically, and many people argue against historicizing ontological conditions in this way. Giddens has in the past argued against the type of historical treatment of embodiment I am advocating, preferring to dehistoricize the experience of embodiment. Pointing to the work of Merleau-Ponty and Goffman, he observes that

> body control is intrinsic to the competent social agent; it is transcultural rather than specifically connected with modernity; and it is a continuous feature of the flow of conduct in the *durée* of daily life. Most importantly, routine control of the body is integral to the very nature both of agency and of being accepted (trusted) by others as competent.
>
> (Giddens 1991: 57)

Giddens subsequently changed his line somewhat, acknowledging that detraditionalization tends to heighten self-awareness (Giddens 1994b). This passage, however, is still a good example of a widespread line of thought which, even if no longer held by Giddens, is certainly propounded by many others. There are two major problems with this type of argument. Firstly, it is unable to account for the fact that while some beliefs and practices are readily able to be reflected upon, others appear as commonsense. Merely drawing attention to them may produce reactions ranging from bemusement at the stupidity of the question to deep anxiety once the practice has been exposed to conscious scrutiny. The second problem with this approach is that it assumes that reflexive awareness is a constant in human societies, whereas on closer inspection it is readily apparent that the extent and character of reflexive awareness vary according to the social formation in question, between social groups within the same society and between individuals. I will return to this second problem in a moment.

Giddens sees the universal nature of such regularized control of the body as the most basic aspect of an 'I/me' differentiation which is universal. That is, in one sense we are the body – when people see us, or when we look at ourselves, we appear as a physical body. At the same time, we have an awareness that we are separate from the body in the sense that we inhabit this body and that we are able to consciously control it. While this is a valid point, Giddens tends to ignore the fact that different social forms constitute the relationship between self and body in different ways. (He only acknowledges any potential for variation in the relationship between 'I' and 'me' in the pathological form of the schizoid character (Giddens 1991: 57–63)). However, somewhat contradictorily, Giddens presents the common argument that with increasing social fragmentation, the body comes to assume a greater role in the constitution of self-identity. This is because when self-identity becomes confused, the body offers a grounding centre for the location of a personal narrative. While reflexive body management and self-care is a basic competency which all people (except the severely disabled) engage in, the nature of these practices varies widely and the level of awareness of these processes can be raised (problematized or disembedded) and lowered (naturalized or habitualized). In the contemporary period the deliberate problematizing and re-habitualization of self-care practices occurs at a much accelerated rate, heightening both self-awareness and ontological insecurity.

In the psychoanalytic tradition, the existence of levels of consciousness is accounted for by the conventional distinction between the non-conscious and unconscious. That which is non-conscious is able to be reflected upon but is normally not thought, while the unconscious realm is repressed and cannot be readily accessed by the person. While there is no substantial difficulty in accessing non-conscious knowledge, the unconscious is more deeply buried, containing much potentially threatening material. The higher levels of consciousness actively repress unconscious knowledge for the sake of the psychological integrity of the person. Of course, in any example there are always different motivations, desires and rationalizations operating on different levels and some are more able to be identified and expressed than others (Sloan 1987). When it comes to theorizing the nature of self-care regimes, the distinction between the non-conscious and the unconscious proves very limited. Psychoanalytic theory deals primarily with the mental status of knowledges, desires, ideas and memories, whereas a theorization of self-care has to account for regularized unconscious acts. What we are concerned with here are those self-care practices which are engaged in unthinkingly and repetitively but cannot be thought, and perhaps have never been reflected upon discursively.

For this purpose Bourdieu's work on belief and the body is invaluable. Bourdieu elaborates the differences between those practices which a person is 'born into' and those which confront the person as distinct entities. To return to the example of language once more, this is the difference between one's mother tongue and a foreign language. When speaking and thinking in one's mother tongue, one is rarely conscious of how this is done. When attempting to learn a foreign language, however, one

> confronts a language that is perceived as such, that is, [...] explicitly consti-
> tuted as such in the form of grammar, rules and exercises, taught by
> institutions expressly designed for that purpose. In the case of primary
> learning, the child learns at the same time to speak the language (which is
> only ever presented in action, in his [*sic*] own or other people's speech) and
> to think *in* (rather than with) the language.
>
> (Bourdieu 1990: 67)

It is apparent then that a very different learning process takes place in each of these cases, and the type of reflection which is possible in relation to the language one speaks is influenced by the way the language was learnt. A person who has learnt a foreign language systematically is more able to reflect explicitly on the way they speak the new language. Their relationship to their new language is more consciously reflective, in that they are aware of the underlying rules and structures of that language. This more abstract understanding may also alter the way they account for their use of their mother tongue, as the same insights can be applied to what they previously were able to do only in practice but not reflect upon in this way. In contrast to the more abstract systematic learning, the mother tongue is a more deeply embedded form of knowledge. The mother tongue has not been mastered through discursive means but has been lived, experienced and absorbed. Bourdieu refers to this type of knowing as practical belief, which, he argues, 'is not a "state of mind", still less an arbitrary adherence to a set of instituted dogmas and doctrines ("beliefs"), but rather a state of the body' (Bourdieu 1990: 68).

This approach is useful to understand the way self-care is practised at the pre-conscious level, or what Marx called 'practical consciousness'. The ways in which one takes care of oneself are enacted through doing what comes naturally or by following commonsense. The means of transmission of these practices is through what Bourdieu refers to as 'practical *mimesis*', which relies on deep iden-tification with the other, and takes place below the level of conscious reflection and expression. He contrasts this with *imitation*, which is a more conscious effort to reproduce an embodied behaviour of an other who is conceived as a model to be emulated (Bourdieu 1993: 73). Mimetic practices are taken on by the person as 'automatic' modes of being, and such self-care regimes lay the foundations for the person's mastery of their own body. This deeply embedded form of self-care, then, is indistinguishable from other taken-for-granted aspects of embodiment such as walking and eating. As Bourdieu points out, through this process of instilling the basic mechanisms of bodily self-control, the values of the society are deeply embodied in its subjects.

> One could endlessly enumerate the values given body, *made* body, by the
> hidden persuasion of an implicit pedagogy which can instill a whole

cosmology, through the injunctions as insignificant as 'sit up straight' or 'don't hold your knife in your left hand', and inscribe the most fundamental principles of the arbitrary content of a culture in seemingly innocuous details of bearing or physical and verbal manners, so putting them beyond the reach of consciousness and explicit statements.

(Bourdieu 1990: 69)

This relationship that one has to one's body is not captured by the psychological terms 'self-concept' or 'self-image', which presuppose a level of conscious reflection which is not apparent in the deepest forms of embodiment. The ontological depth of mimetic self-care practices is often underestimated by writers who attach no significance to the level of integration through which self-care practices are constituted. It is worth quoting Bourdieu one last time in relation to this difference:

So long as the work of education is not clearly institutionalized as a specific, autonomous practice, so long as it is the whole group and a whole symbolically structured environment, without specialized agents or specific occasions, that exerts an anonymous, diffuse pedagogic action, the essential part of the *modus operandi* that defines practical mastery is transmitted through practice, in the practical state, without rising to the level of discourse.

(Bourdieu 1990: 73–4)

Such transmission of deeply embedded self-care practices through practical mimesis is the result of prolonged mutual co-presence. However, when education is conducted by 'specialized agents' in the 'specific occasions' characteristic of professional-institutional integration, it is communicated at the level of discursive consciousness, requiring the more conscious and active process of learning. I will use the term 'active self-care' to refer to these more self-conscious and more calculating self-care practices, as distinct from the relatively taken-for-granted character of more embedded self-care practices.

Let us consider the type of relation with the body which is associated with the disembodied, or technologically mediated, level of integration. Disembodied self-care promotion inevitably operates at a higher level of reflexive consciousness than more embedded self-care practices, at least as it is presented in the first point of delivery. As such, not only is there a difference in the content of the self-care knowledge or skills being communicated, but, at a more fundamental level, it involves a much more active relationship between the actor and their body. Without the ongoing physical presence of the other, in this case the producer of self-care advice, the audience member cannot absorb the message through practical mimesis. He or she must be open to persuasion, willing to act on the advice provided, and must be able to consciously integrate this new self-care practice into their existing lifestyle. Discursively constituted practices often come to be re-embedded over time. Through routinized repetition a practice can drop from the person's conscious mind to the level of practical consciousness, or, in more popular terms, after a while it becomes 'second nature'. The first time a person flosses their teeth in response to advice from their dentist, partner or television, it seems an awkward and silly thing to be doing. If that person was to repeat the procedure every night for a few months, they would likely feel uneasy about going to bed with 'dirty' teeth if they neglected to floss and would find themselves flossing 'automatically' without having consciously to remind themselves to do so. This form of re-embedding occurs through repetition, but there is also another type of re-embedding engaged in by self-care promoters. In order for a novel practice to be received by an audience as a 'sensible' modification of one's existing self-care practices, self-care promoters often attempt to describe their novel self-care practices as a continuation of accepted or embedded practices. The New Age movement has been at the forefront of producing and marketing novel self-care practices which respond to the need to authenticate the highly self-conscious manipulation of one's self-identity, usually by casting the new identity or behaviour as more 'natural' than the taken-for-granted practices they seek to replace. In the next chapter, I will argue that the appeal to nature and tradition in alternative therapies says more about the ontological dimension of contemporary self-care practices than it does about the content of the therapies which make such claims.

Despite the re-embedding of self-care practices over time, the cumulative effect of contemporary self-care promotion has been the perpetual disembedding and re-embedding of self-care practices across smaller and smaller time-frames. The process of changing the health behaviour of a target audience usually involves drawing their attention to their current practices, alerting them to the 'hidden dangers', then proposing a 'safer' alternative. From that point on, if the communication has fulfilled its objectives, the audience will feel guilty engaging in what they now know to be risky behaviour or else choose the guilt-free alternative. Ontological security rests on a foundation of deeply held beliefs and practices which can be relied upon and trusted (Giddens 1991: 38). In Bourdieu's words, 'It is because agents never know completely what they are doing that what they do has more sense than they will ever know' (Bourdieu 1990: 69). One's ontological security is predicated on such a belief that the most taken-for-granted aspects of one's self and the world are true and that continued faith in such assumptions will ensure safety from risks. The perpetual disembedding of health beliefs and self-care practices can, however, undermine ontological security by repeatedly problematizing previously taken-for-granted aspects of one's self-identity and lifestyle.

Modernity has transformed the relatively stable and constraining social contexts of the pre-modern world into what appear to be increasingly open fields of action. Whereas in social forms framed by the dominance of face-to-face integration, a person was born into a pre-determined place in the social order governed by comparatively taken-for-granted cultural norms, in a social form framed by looser and more abstract integrative mechanisms, the contemporary individual must create their own tenuous foothold in the shifting sands of a more uncertain social sphere. In earlier periods, this individualization was the condition of life for a privileged few, but during the twentieth century this condition spread throughout the whole of late capitalist societies. Rather than being a choice, individualization is unavoidable. As Ulrich Beck and Elisabeth Beck-Gernsheim put it:

> Individualization is a compulsion, albeit a paradoxical one, to create, to stage-manage, not only one's biography but the bonds and networks surrounding it, and to do this amid changing preferences and at successive stages of life, while constantly adapting to the conditions of the labour market, the education system, the welfare state, etc.
>
> (Beck and Beck-Gernsheim 1996: 27)

These are 'precarious freedoms' where the possibilities and responsibilities of choice have been imposed upon the person, forcing them to act. With this detraditionalization have come many new techniques for the constitution of self-identity in more abstract ways which fill the void left by the erosion of the informal cultural reproduction of subjectivity.

3 Sending the health message

> Would you like a quick, sure-fire recipe for handling worrying situations – a technique you can start using right away, before you go any further in reading this book? [...] I got it from Mr Carrier personally when we were having lunch together one day at the Engineer's club in New York.
>
> Dale Carnegie, *How to Stop Worrying and Start Living* (1962: 30)

There is nothing unusual about the aptly named Mr Carrier passing advice on to Dale Carnegie over lunch one day. What is novel, historically, is that Dale Carnegie would write this advice down, cobbled together with dozens of other snippets, and publish the results as a book. Dale Carnegie's genius was to realize that, with the right approach and packaging, such mundane fragments of popular wisdom gleaned can satisfy some popular craving. As the writer of some of the first best-selling self-help books, Carnegie helped shape a genre of publishing composed of advice that was previously communicated orally as everyday conversation topics between friends and family.

This chapter explores the growth of such disembodied health advice in mediated communications, including self-help books, websites and advertising. I am not interested in the content of the advice, however. I don't know whether Aitkins' diet is better than Pritikan's, or what happens when governments tell elderly citizens to be more active. These are interesting questions, and discussion of the merits of such advice fills millions of published pages and millions of broadcast hours around the world every year. But it is not that I think that the overall quantity of advice is increasing; in any case, it is impossible to measure the total quantity of information individuals receive from all sources. It is clear, though, that the proportion of information and advice that comes to individuals through mediated communications has increased dramatically in a few generations, and that the more abstract forms of communication are now culturally dominant, in that the information they convey tends to reconstitute and replace the information produced and communicated by individuals themselves. What interests me is the cumulative impact of this growth in mediated discussion, advice and encouragement. I do not deal here with disembodied interpersonal communication such as letter writing, telephone conversations and email correspondence, where there is an ongoing conversation between two people, but will instead focus on mass communication such as books, newspapers, television and multimedia, where the flow of information is generally in one direction.

It seems that most of the health advice we hear goes in one ear and out the other most of the time. The current consensus is that mediated messages have little lasting impact on people's health beliefs and practices. While mass media may be useful in increasing public awareness of health issues in the short term, media campaigns alone are thought to be generally ineffective in changing self-care behaviour (Flora and Wallack 1990). Even the best-researched and focus-group tested anti-smoking television commercials seem to have little impact in themselves. Where they have been used extensively, they have not had any appreciable effect on smoking rates. Instead, smoking rates declined steadily at around one per cent per annum irrespective of when and how often the ads were screened (Duckett 1997). When governments try to change self-care practices, the 'productive' power of mass media campaigns is usually complemented with the 'restrictive' power of legislative action. In the case of tobacco, this has involved running health advertising campaigns in conjunction with legal measures preventing smoking in workplaces and restaurants, increasing tobacco taxes and restricting the supply of cigarettes to minors. When health information is included in entertainment programming in programmes such as the long-running American hospital drama *ER*, a similar pattern is evident. A recent study surveyed different groups of regular *ER* viewers about health issues that were featured in the programme's storylines. Different viewers were polled before an issue was dealt with in the programme, shortly afterwards, and others were polled months later. Immediately after an episode was screened, *ER* viewers were more informed than they were before, but several months later they had the same level of familiarity and understanding of the issues as they did before the programme was screened (Brodie *et al.* 2001).

While the specific impact of any one health message seems negligible, the cumulative impact has been immense. At the level of the individual, as Alberto Melucci observed, the proliferation of sources of information requires that 'individuals and groups must possess a certain degree of autonomy and formal capacities for learning and acting that enable them to function as reliable, self-regulating units' (Melucci 1994: 101). Health behaviour is now shaped less by restrictive regulation of behaviour than by productive interference in the cognitive and motivational processes of individuals. The shaping of self-care through contemporary mass communications has changed the actor's relationship to their body and their self, ushering in a more self-active and self-conscious form of subjectivity.

The dominance of disembodied forms of interaction is one of the conditions contributing to a more reflexive or self-conscious form of subjectivity in postmodern societies. As John Thompson has argued, with the growth of mediated interaction, 'the capacity to experience was increasingly disconnected from the activity of encountering' (Thompson 1996: 97). People can know in more detail what it feels like to be in someone else's shoes. Every television viewer has 'experienced' dozens of bank robberies, hundreds of car chases and thousands of murders. The depictions of these events may be unrepresentative and superficial but nevertheless their cumulative effect is to create an air of familiarity with extreme events. When people come to experience those events first-hand, a common response is summed up in the sentiment 'I never thought it would happen to *me*', which is a feature of any postmodern survivor story. This is the experience not of being in an unfamiliar experience, but of finding oneself in a situation which is very familiar but which the person thought they would never experience themselves.

To extend this observation to the inner life of the person, we should also note that the world of the postmodern subject is saturated with mediated images and accounts of other people's self-conduct, self-formation and self-problematization. This is most starkly illustrated in daytime chat shows such as *Oprah* and *Donahue*, but is a feature of virtually all drama, especially 'soap operas'. This is also a strong element in the appeal of celebrities. The audience follow the 'behind-the-scenes' dramas in the personal lives of media celebrities. They share a particular form of intimacy with the celebrity, which Thompson describes as a 'non-recip-rocal intimacy at a distance' (Thompson 1996: 99). Despite the shallowness of this intimacy compared with face-to-face reciprocal relationships, the trials and tribulations of media celebrities are often experienced with some intensity by audiences. The death of Princess Diana, the most extreme recent example of this phenomenon, was experienced by a huge proportion of the populations of English-speaking countries as if they had lost a personal friend. Through drama, chat shows and celebrity watching, postmodern audiences have considerable insights into other people's self-management and self-formation.

In the examples given above, the audience become more readily able to reflect on their own emotional situation and their own active self-management because they have seen and heard many others express their own thoughts on such matters. With regard to the physical appearance of the body, a similar argu-ment can be made that the proliferation of images of the body has resulted in a heightened reflexive awareness of one's own physical appearance. Images of beautiful others became widespread in women's magazines early in the twentieth century, and have continuously expanded since with the advent of film and tele-vision. With the availability of cheap photographic equipment and now video, individuals go through life seeing images of themselves in everyday life and at significant events. As Featherstone notes, the proliferation of images invites comparison and reflection, providing the individual with constant reminders of what they are and what they might become. The resulting focus on image has fostered the emergence of the 'performing self' who places greater emphasis on appearance, display and the management of impressions (Featherstone 1991).

These have been the principal effects on the consumers of information. On the other side, focusing on the production of health advice, the most obvious effect has been the enormous power that is available to those who seek to shape the way individuals exercise their freedom to care for themselves. The size of audiences and markets is increased as communications technology with global reach creates enormous economies of scale. Governments, corporations and other actors now have the capacity to reach much deeper into the constitution of subjectivity than they have ever had before.

These books will change your life

Self-help books now constitute a large proportion of books sold, and non-fiction best-seller lists usually include several self-help titles dealing with relationships, diet and personal finance. Their popularity became obvious during the 1970s, ringing alarm bells for intellectuals such as Richard Sennett and Christopher Lasch, who saw the growth of the genre as evidence of moral decay. James Lincoln Collier points to the appearance of self-help books on the *New York Times* best-sellers in the 1970s as evidence for his thesis that selfishness is on the rise in America:

> In 1971, *The Sensuous Man* and *Any Woman Can!* made the list. In the summer of 1973 *Dr Atkins' Diet Revolution*, *The Joy of Sex*, and *I'm OK–You're OK* were on the list together. In 1975 Sylvia Porter's *Money Book*, *Power! Winning Through Intimidation*, *The Relaxation Response*, *The Save Your Life Diet*, and *TM* were on simultaneously.
>
> (Collier 1991: 232)

For intellectuals, who frequent bookshops but are not regular watchers of daytime television or readers of women's magazines, these books were the first visible evidence of a radical cultural change that was quickly labelled narcissistic. These reactions will be considered in Chapter 7, but here I will sketch out some key issues in the historical development of health-related self-help books, and some of the common features of many contemporary self-help books that evoke such strong responses from intellectuals and such demand from consumers.

Before the late eighteenth century, self-help books had very little impact on proactive self-care practices in any society. The earliest example of a successful comprehensive popularization of contemporary medical knowledge in English was William Buchan's *Domestic Medicine*, published in Edinburgh in 1769. It was immediately successful, being reprinted extensively in Britain and America. Buchan's book was not intended to replace the physician's role, but informed wealthy readers how to complement their medical care with sound self-care techniques. This self-help book, like other literature, was at that time affordable to only the wealthiest part of the population. Buchan encouraged the charitable among his readership to help the poor and illiterate with the knowledge they had gained, lest the illiterate be dependent on ignorant and superstitious quacks. Compared with present-day self-help books, these texts had a very small readership confined to the aristocracy and educated middle classes (Blake 1977).

Through the nineteenth century in America and Europe, 'domestic medicine' texts sought to complement professional treatment by providing current medical advice to those unable to see a practitioner or who preferred to treat themselves. These books were not focused on preventive care, but were almost solely concerned with self-treatment of ailments and illnesses. Their form was usually similar to that of a cookbook, with instructions and procedures for self-treatment using the same techniques and the same medicines as were used by doctors, which were widely available. American self-help texts responded to the shortage of physicians in rural areas, believing that the promulgation of medical knowledge in such circumstances would serve to heighten appreciation for academically trained physicians and teach the reading public how to avoid the quacks who might take advantage of such a medical shortage (Blake 1977: 15–16). Whereas British domestic medical texts appear to be directed at a smaller and more educated audience, American self-help books are more often directed at the rural poor. This was likely due to higher rates of literacy in the Bible-reading Protestant United States. It may also have been because the experience of migrating to the colonies created a rupture in the handing-down of traditional forms of self-care and folk remedies. Folk health-care systems such as herbalism seem to have endured much longer in the more traditional European societies, whereas the relatively individualistic and modern settler societies were more fertile grounds for the formulation of both reflexive self-care practices and novel systems of expert care.

Other early titles included John Tennent's *Every Man His Own Doctor, or The Poor Planter's Physician*, which went through five editions between 1734 and 1737 (L. Levin *et al.* 1979). Another influential example from this period was *Primitive Physick*, written by the Methodist John Wesley and published in London in 1747 and Philadelphia in 1764. Wesley decried the abstraction of health care – from a set of cures handed down from father to son (or, more likely, mother to daughter), medicine had become a mystified and exotic body of knowledge out of reach of ordinary people. Many of these self-help books were critical of the professionalization of medicine and encouraged lay people to educate themselves in order to become their own doctors, following an American tradition of staunch self-reliance. They spoke the language of a medical reformation in which the doctors represented the clergy standing between the individual and their godly body. Taking the place of the doctor/priest was the book. These domestic medicine books aimed to provide easily available solutions to a range of conditions, able to be practised by any person without the aid of professional intervention (Blake 1977: 18–19). While these self-help texts may have promised to overcome the abstraction of medical practice by providing popularly accessible do-it-yourself alternatives, they were abstract in a different way. While the provider and recipient of advice in a professional encounter may be speaking different languages, they are at least in the same room. The writer and reader of a self-help text have a more abstract relationship in that they are separated by time and space and can know very little of the other's circumstances. The self-help book may be readable but it is of necessity simplistic, for the writer must write for a generic imaginary audience.

One of the most popular of the vast array of nineteenth-century American domestic medicine books was J.C. Gunn's *Domestic Medicine, or Poor Man's Friend*. Gunn repeated a widespread religious critique of professionalization, preferring the substances which God had 'stored in our mountains, fields and meadows' over the expensive and imported man-made concoctions favoured by medicine. He complained that professionals used language

> to conceal the naked poverty and bareness of the sciences. [...] if the great mass of the people knew how much pains were taken by scientific men, to throw dust in their eyes by the use of ridiculous high-sounding terms [...] mankind would soon be undeceived, as to the little difference that really exists between themselves and the *very learned* portion of the community.
>
> (cited in Blake 1977: 20)

An example of Gunn's self-reliant approach is his opinion that any person with firmness and average dexterity could amputate a limb, a view repeated in A.C. Goodlett's *Family Physician* in 1838, which promises that 'any man, unless he is an idiot or an absolute fool, can perform this operation' (cited in Blake 1977: 25). These anti-intellectual and anti-medical approaches to the popularization of knowledge aimed to translate current medical knowledge into commonsense, but despite this oppositional approach, the self-care practices they advocated were not very different from the pro-medical texts of the time, both reflecting America's preoccupation with harsh 'heroic' treatments.

Early twentieth-century medical self-help books were directed at an audience which had more ready access to medical services and in which there was a much greater faith in the therapeutic capacities of doctors. Rather than providing simplified medical textbooks for those without access to a doctor, these new texts provided a general introduction to health and disease with limited self-help advice, restricted to hygiene and emergency first aid (Blake 1977: 28). Typical of its kind was a forty-eight-page booklet published in the US by the Mutual Benefit Health and Accident Association and called *What to Do Until the Doctor Comes* (Clarfield 1997). A much more comprehensive text was Fishbein's *Modern Home Medical Adviser*, first published in 1935 and selling over one million copies. The author describes his book as 'in a way a modern substitute for the old-time family medicine book that along with the Bible used to be on the table of sitting rooms in many a home in the United States'. The *Modern Home Medical Adviser* is characteristic of early twentieth-century medical self-help books in that rather than instructing the reader how to be their own doctor, it instead explains to the reader how physicians treat disease. Fishbein wanted to communicate 'in a modern manner what every intelligent person ought to know about scientific medicine and hygiene' (cited in Blake 1977: 11). From the early twentieth century up to the late 1960s, most health self-help books played down the importance of self-treatment, instead encouraging professional consultation for all but the most minor complaints. With their firm faith in modern medical care, these books played down the importance of self-care. Their purpose was instead to make people more at ease with medical practices, to build a receptive and compliant public for the expansion of medical dominance over health care (Willis 1989).

Throughout the twentieth century an increasing proportion of the population learnt an increasing proportion of their techniques for self-care from printed matter. Compared with the nineteenth century the volume of sales is now enormous, and self-help books now comprise a much larger proportion of the publishing industry. Between the early 1980s and the early 1990s the number of self-help books selling over 50,000 copies in the United States had more than doubled from below ten to around twenty per year (J. Ryan *et al.* 1994). The range of topics covered by contemporary self-care books is much more extensive and the texts themselves tend to assume a higher level of medical knowledge in their audience (L. Levin *et al.* 1979: 22).

While self-help books are more visible to intellectuals who browse in bookstores, and were the object of much of the criticism that I will discuss in later chapters, the proliferation of health advice found in magazines, television and radio is more inescapable. At least since the turn of the twentieth century, magazines, especially those aimed at women, have commonly included self-help advice of various sorts, and the advice offered in these magazines has tended to follow the intellectual trends of the day (Cancian and Gordon 1988). In the 1970s many self-care magazines focusing on mental, emotional and physical well-being were launched in the United States. In the hey-day of popular psychology, *Psychology Today, American Health, Prevention* and *Self* each had a circulation of over one million copies (Glassner 1989: 180).

Health information is routinely reported in the news, which familiarizes people with scientific determinations on healthy behaviour. Consider these articles, which are all taken from a single issue of Melbourne's largest circulation daily newspaper, the *Herald Sun*, on 15 October 1997:

Heroin a $2.9b growth industry

Victoria has up to 20,000 heroin addicts, contributing to the drug's estimated growth industry in Australia.

Mature women shun body woes

Middle aged women are not generally worried about their body shape despite the effects of menopause, new research shows.

Rail inquest safety plea

Bright yellow warning lines will be painted at railway crib crossings to alert pedestrians to the danger of walking into the path of approaching trains.

More steal to gamble

Nearly a third of problem gamblers seeking help for their addiction have admitted turning to crime, figures revealed.

Children in calls for affection

Children yearned for more affection and understanding from their parents at a time when family relationships were under increasing pressure, a new survey shows.

Stress can stunt growth

Stress caused by family conflict including parents' divorce or separation can stunt a child's growth, according to new research.

Baby bug asthma link

A sexually transmitted bacterium which infects unborn babies could lead to childhood asthma.

Every day the news media run dozens of such reports detailing the results of health research and treatment innovations. The articles above are not part of a health update special or a lifestyle section but appeared in the general news section. It is no longer possible to argue that the general public do not have access to health information. We are in fact bombarded by such information. However, most such health reports give minimal practical advice, and even when they do touch on self-care practices, they do so in a cursory and often confusing manner. It is impossible for any person to keep abreast of all such information, let alone put it into practice in their lives. This creates a feeling that there is always more that one could do to take care of oneself – by taking more notice of such information, making further enquiries and by changing one's behaviour in a more concerted fashion in response to the latest findings. But because the flow of information is so overwhelming, if a person was to take all such recommendations seriously, their self-care practices would constantly be in a state of flux.

Producing more exciting self-help books: New Age hyper-individualism

The New Age movement, which grew out of the spiritual arm of the counter-culture, has been a major influence in shaping popular understandings of the rise of self-care since the 1970s, viewing this as a sign that Western societies are entering an era of heightened spiritual maturity. While many New Age writers discuss psychical evolution, Theodore Roszak's *Unfinished Animal: The Aquarian Frontier and the Evolution of Consciousness* is perhaps the most developed example of this notion. Roszak, who was part of the counter-cultural 'spiritual awakening', sees self-awareness as a by-product of profound historical change and a promising shift away from nineteenth-century values centred on competition to a culture of cooperative self-fulfilment:

We can discern, through all these starry-eyed images of an Aquarian Age filled with wonders and wellbeing, a transformation of human personality in progress which is of *evolutionary* proportions, a shift of consciousness fully as epoch-making as the appearance of speech or of the tool-making talents in our cultural repertory.

(Roszak 1975: 3)

For Roszak, the growth in reflexive practices was evolutionary because it involved an innovation which was 'prophetic, ingeniously "adaptive" and apt to become species-wide', marking 'collective arrival at a new stage of being' (Roszak 1975: 76). This is an overtly idealist conception of a pre-ordained human destiny, which, due to historical circumstances, is close to being realized. The New Age movement thus sees the contemporary interest in self-care as part of a broader collective spiritual evolution of consciousness which centres on self-exploration and self-transformation. Roszak believes that humanity has moved onto the next level, and from this point on must be seen 'no longer as *homo faber* or *homo economicus*, but as humanity transcendent, seeker of meaning, creator of visions' (Roszak 1975: 79). The New Age movement thus celebrates introspection as a primary virtue and as the defining feature of humanity's next phase.

Despite the appeal to those devotees of reflexive spiritual practice who would like to think that they are at the leading edge of the evolution of the species, there is no reason why the satisfaction of the material requirements of life should necessarily lead to an interest in such questions of self-identity. There is no clear relationship between levels of economic well-being and levels of religiosity. Also, this evolutionary explanation does not explain the specific character of the new forms of spiritual practice – their preoccupation with the sacralization of the inner self or their belief in nature as an ultimate measure of value.

A common New Age explanation for the rise of the new awareness is that it stems from technological advances (the products of intellect) catching up with the innate spiritual potentials of human beings. At last we have created a material world which allows us to express our untapped potential. In the 1930s a number of writers set about integrating popular understandings of physics with Asian mysticism and Western occult traditions. These were synthesizing works which attempted to demonstrate a convergence between these radically different intellectual traditions. One of these compendiums of scientific and mystical convergence, Vera Stanley Alder's 1938 book *The Finding of the Third Eye*, projects a future in which technological developments will enhance the spiritual evolution of the species:

The earliest results achieved will be, firstly, a considerable improvement and control of health and good looks, a growing capacity for happiness, an inability to worry or fear; a gaining of popularity, and freedom from boredom. In time, when greater strides are made, there will be immunity from disease, conquering of fatigue, and prolonging of youth. There will be a growing capacity for helping others, a mastery of sorrow and pain, and the development of healing power. A growing inner force will be felt, both for creating ideas and the carrying of them out.

(Alder 1968: 24)

Alder writes about the super-man within us, arguing: 'On every hand we find clues to the strange and tremendous forces hidden within us, forces that when properly understood and developed could certainly lead us to unimaginable power and achievement' (Alder 1968: 22). There is a potential power and omnipotence which is every person's birthright.

> There is nothing to prove that we could not all attain complete mastery over our lives and fortunes, and reach ideal happiness, were we given this key, and had the will and the determination to use it. Had we this secret, instead of being, as we are, slaves to life, to our possessions, our environment, ill health, 'bad luck' and the rest, we could be master and controller of all our circumstances, and welcome with content and understanding everything that life brings to us.
>
> (Alder 1968: 22–3)

This theme has been echoed by numerous more recent New Age writers, who place greater emphasis particularly on communication technologies. Barbara Marx Hubbard, a prominent New Age writer, for example, believes that technologies of mass communication (televisions, telephones, satellites, computers) are extending our planetary nervous system, allowing us to tune in spiritually to the health of all parts of the earth (Hubbard 1991: 7). In the New Age belief system there is a hidden deeper level of reality which underlies and explains all observable phenomena (Ziguras 1997b). In the past this was held to be only accessible through altered or enhanced states of consciousness, but increasingly New Age writers speak of this enlightenment occurring at the level of populations, facilitated by electronic communications. The result is a 'democratizing awareness' to which each of us is entitled. The consequences of this communication-led evolution of consciousness are profound, as Hubbard explains:

> We will either stumble blindly towards self-destruction through misuse of our new powers, or we will move consciously toward a new order of the ages. We will begin the great evolutionary tasks: the restoration of the earth, the freeing of people from want, the development of the vast untapped potential of our bodyminds, and the exploration of the unlimited frontiers of outer space.
>
> (Hubbard 1991: 5)

Like many other New Age writers, Hubbard argues that what had once been experienced as mystical insight, the sudden blinding enlightenment, such as St Paul received on the road to Damascus, is now becoming the norm. This she refers to as the democratization of awareness: 'As we intersect as a planetary whole, each person is becoming a clearer channel to the "Source", the Process of evolution, God' (Hubbard 1991: 6). The New Age has a globalized sense of humanity as a planetary whole which is partly an expression of an ecological consciousness but also the self-understanding of those who feel part of a global community in which each of its members is connected by copper wires and the free flow of information.

The central preoccupations of this literature on awareness are the increased ability to take control of one's self, to see through ideology, to throw off shackles of the past. The New Age movement provides tools with which people can see through the taken-for-granted aspects of their beliefs and behaviours, and with which they can rebuild themselves in the desired way. It promises empowerment by claiming that the self is malleable and that people can rebuild themselves through introspection and self-transformation. In practice, however, the New Age succumbs to the problems of solipsism and cognitivism identified earlier because it lacks an understanding of the social and psychological constraints on reflexive action.

Louise Hay's best-selling book *You Can Heal Your Life* (1988) was for a few years treated like a bible by many New Agers. The author had cured herself of cancer after coming to understand what she saw as the metaphysical causes of the disease. She extrapolated her findings about the emotional and psychical bases of illness to other complaints and many people listened. According to Hay, bladder problems meant you were 'pissed off with life' and eye problems meant that you were trying to avoid seeing something. She advised her readers to try to cure illnesses by repeating affirmations to themselves – positive thoughts which would replace the negative mental energy and eliminate the related physical symptoms. A former devotee of Louise Hay describes the health-beliefs which went along with this book, and others of the period:

> Thanks to *You Can Heal Your Life*, many of us experienced an important shift towards taking more responsibility for our physical and emotional health and appreciating the undoubted impact of mind on body. But the cult of Louise eventually grew to have a dark side. It became too easy to simplistically put a label on someone's pain and glibly toss off a wordy remedy to make it all better.
>
> (Ackroyd 1997: 24)

All that was needed to remain perfectly healthy, according to these writers, was a strong and focused will. The message was that good health is completely within reach of the striving individual – we can all be perfectly fit and well if we just set our minds to it. This is an ideology of autonomy in which the individual is portrayed as free to be whatever he or she wants to be. These proponents of complete personal responsibility will tolerate no discussion of the constraints on reflexive action. For Louise Hay, physical reality is a projection of the mind, and to blame an illness on factors beyond one's control is seen as a way of avoiding responsibility for one's own condition.

Hay's best-seller was perhaps the most outlandish of a swag of books and magazine articles extolling the virtues of positive thinking for health, and especially for cancer treatment. Titles such as *The Power of Positive Thinking, The A–Z of Positive Thinking* and *Fighting Spirit* advocated the use of affirmations such as 'my cancer cells are dissolving', and 'I am a powerful person capable of healing myself'. These notions were taken up by television news and current affairs reporters keen for good-news stories who would explain how an individual triumphed over a life-threatening condition by virtue of their strength of character, determination and faith. As Sue Wilkinson and Celia Kitzinger (2000) have shown, such messages have profoundly affected patients' ways of dealing with serious illness, to the extent that most patients now feel obliged to 'think positive'. Thinking positive now functions as a socially normative moral requirement, representing an expected pattern of patient behaviour (appearing cheerful, motivated and optimistic) rather than referring to the patient's internal cognitive state.

After a run of big-selling self-help books in the 1980s, including Hay's, the self-improvement publishing industry became increasingly lucrative and competitive. In order to make their books stand out from the crowd on shelves of the personal growth section, authors and publishers became ever more extravagant in their claims. Ackroyd remembers:

> Motivational authors sailed off into a ocean of hyperbole. A flotilla of tomes appeared with such titles as *Absolute Happiness, Ageless Body, Super Self, Total Prosperity, Boundless Energy, The Sky's the Limit,* (inevitably) *You Can Have It All!* and even *Absolutely, Positively the Last Self-Help Book You'll Ever Need to Read.*
> (Ackroyd 1997: 24)

Through the 1980s a subculture emerged in which it was believed that 'you create your own reality' and where the phrase 'that's your reality' was used as a justification for dishonesty and indifference to the suffering of others (Ziguras 1997b). The sick were sick because of their state of mind and the poor were poor because of their poverty of consciousness. According to the New Age ontology dominant in this subculture, both the self and reality outside the self are completely mutable – the observable world is energy shaped into physical form by thought. That is, the physical world, like Star Trek's holodeck, is merely a surface which masks the unstable reality underneath. Starhawk, one of the most prominent feminist New Age writers, sees the physical world as formed by energy in the same way as stalactites are formed by dropping water:

> If we cause a change in the energy patterns, they in turn will cause a change in the physical world – just as, if we change the course of an underground river, new series of stalactites will be formed in new veins of rock
> (Starhawk 1979: 183)

The appearance of fixity of selves and objects should not be taken too seriously, since underneath at a deeper level of reality all is fluid and changeable by will. At this deeper level,

> all things are swirls of energy, vortexes of moving forces, currents in an ever-changing sea. Underlying the appearance of separateness, of fixed objects within a linear stream of time, reality is a field of energies that congeal, temporarily, into forms. In time, all 'fixed' things dissolve, only to coalesce again into new forms, new vehicles.
>
> (Starhawk 1979: 181)

For this reason, goddess-worshipping women prefer to employ powerful rituals which work directly on the underlying flow of energy instead of pursuing more conventional forms of social empowerment, much to the dismay of more materialist feminists (Denfeld 1995). The practice of using will or imagination to change reality is sometimes referred to as creative visualization. Shakti Gawain, in her seminal work on the subject, explains how creative visualization works:

> Our physical universe is not really composed of any 'matter' at all; its basic component is a kind of force or essence which we call *energy*. [...] Thought is a quick, light, mobile form of energy. It manifests instantaneously, unlike the denser forms such as matter. [...] The idea is like a blueprint; it creates an image of the form, which then magnetizes and guides the physical energy to flow into that form and eventually manifests it on the physical plane.
>
> (Gawain 1982: 5–6)

This ontology supports a radically idealist and voluntaristic attitude towards one's health. Starhawk does, however, have sufficient political understanding to acknowledge that the New Age idea that we create our own reality 'can only conceivably make sense to white upper-middle-class Americans, and then only some of the time' (Starhawk 1990: 37). And while the politicized wing of the New Age acknowledges that 'reality also has the power to shape us', a politics based purely on a 'psychology of liberation', as Starhawk describes her own endeavours, can conceive of collective ritual but not collective political action to tackle the social and environmental causes of illness. Ackroyd sees this as a form of New Age fascism in which only the positive would be tolerated, forcing the repression of concerns about powers greater than the self under feelings of defeat and shame (Ackroyd 1997). What is motivating this culture is a desire to transcend the limitations imposed by the human condition. An age-old desire perhaps, but never before has it been so naïvely proposed by so many. Ackroyd describes it as a desire for a 'get-out-of-the-human-condition-free card', which is deeply entrenched in a culture which sees no limits to technological advancement: 'We are the generation who refused to accept the limitations endured by our ancestors. We wanted more and we made damn sure we got it. Now we want it all. We want it easily and we want it yesterday' (Ackroyd 1997: 26). Of course many readers were not able to change unpleasant aspects of themselves or their lives, even after reading dozens of self-help books which had told them how easy these tasks should be.

Another New Ager who mastered the commercial exploitation of the desire for quick and easy self-transformation was Master Charles. His 'genius' was to realize that what he and other devotees had actually been doing during the years they had spent in an ashram while performing Vedic rituals, meditating and chanting was to use mantras to rescript their databases. He concluded that the psychic effects of caves, long noted by high-country yogis, are actually due to the correspondence and harmonizing of the cave's echo interval with certain brain-wave frequencies. Master Charles (formerly Brother Charles) left the ashram and set about producing a shortcut to nirvana in the form of a series of audiotapes which exploit the consciousness-altering properties of certain frequencies in a more convenient manner. Master Charles claims to have accelerated traditional spiritual growth by 75 per cent, boasting 'we've got the cave experience of fifty years down to twelve – that's a big breakthrough!' (cited in Hooper and Teresi 1990: 168). In doing so he developed 'contemporary high-tech meditation' and founded an organization he called Multidimensional Synchronicity Through Holodynamics to spread the word, the tapes and the seminars. 'After all', he says, 'we are Americans. We have created McDonald's. If we can create fast foods, can we not create fast enlightenment?' (cited in Hooper and Teresi 1990: 71).

The point of these examples is to demonstrate the types of claims about the radical mutability of the self which are routinely made at the individualistic end of the self-help spectrum. As Ackroyd points out, the intense competition in the self-help industry leads to an exaggeration of the power of the self-transforma-tion product being marketed. These individualistic forms of self-care promotion exist within and feed a New Age subculture in which audiences are often already well versed in the philosophies and self-enhancement practices of the particular genre. The passages by Starhawk quoted above do not look so unusual when placed alongside the many other New Age neo-feminist texts on the market which espouse similar messages and when located in the context of the broader New Age neo-feminist self-help culture (Sethna 1992). A striking example of such a radical individualistic self-empowerment subculture is the extropian movement, a Californian self-empowerment subculture which embraces tech-nology to fight bodily decay. Explaining extropian principles, Romana Machado (1994) warns her readers on the Web :

> Action is necessary, because 'rust never sleeps.' If you do nothing, personal entropy wins. Entropy is a measure of increasing disorder, a force of nature that opposes the life of each person, driving all dullness, depression, disease, death and decay. Personal entropy is your sworn, sleepless enemy. There is much that each person can do, privately, to win against it.

The extropians believe you can fight personal entropy by maximizing personal extropy through aggressive self-improvement. Machado urges her readers to begin right away using all available technologies. 'You can combat personal entropy now, with a campaign for personal enhancement through applied technology and hard science.' She identifies five spheres of the self which need caring for: your mind, your body, your financial security, your personal power and your body after death. (The last is achieved with cryogenic suspension.)

For extropians, self-transformation involves actively enhancing every aspect of one's self in order to be better than others and better than one's present self. Max More (1997), in an article advocating technological self-transformation, argues that a 'commitment to self-transformation means a refusal to acquiesce in mediocrity, a questioning of limits to one's potential, and a drive to perpetually overcome psychological, social, physiological, genetic, and neurological constraints'. By 'social constraints', More is referring to people who have the potential to hinder their self-improvement campaign. In their preoccupation with a hyper-individuated self-transformation which advocates withdrawing from interpersonal relationships in order to better look after oneself, the extropians are an extreme example of what Hochschild (1994) refers to as 'cool' self-help. Unlike 'warm' self-help advice, which attempts to help the reader to build strong interpersonal relationships, they repeatedly affirm the importance of establishing increased independence and detachment from others.

These three philosophies of self-care promotion expounded by the lifestyle health promoters, the New Right and the New Age movement obviously differ from each other in many ways but all exaggerate the capacity for reflexive action to improve the health of the individual. They promote self-care in such a way as to make the individual think that their social situation and their health status is of their own making. By overstating individual agency, they lay blame on the sick for their illnesses and the poor for their poverty. By overstating the freedom of the individual to re-create their identity, behaviour and conditions of life, they deliver disappointment to those whose attempts at self-transformation fail because they lack a reflexivity as to the social contexts which shape their health and their self-care practices.

Over the course of the 1980s and 1990s, New Age therapies and health advice gained mainstream credibility, and these self-transformative techniques became popular in management training, particularly in the United States. While 'alternative' New Agers who have retained a counter-cultural opposition to mainstream lifestyles consider the 'external' trappings of consumerism as unhealthy distractions from inner happiness, mainstream New Agers often treat success in the market as expressive of an inner godliness, in much the same way as those early capitalists who were the subject of Weber's classic study (Heelas 1992, 1996). Success in work and material wealth are revered not in themselves but as signs of general well-being, of being in touch with one's inner self and therefore able to control one's material reality at will. Heelas (1992) argues that the cultural contradiction Daniel Bell (1976) describes between the cultural demands for self-realization and systemic need for rational organizational is able to be overcome in the mainstream New Age by spiritualizing the rewards of working life, finding meaning by interpreting conventional materialism through the filter of an inward-looking religiosity.

At the same time as this transformation has taken place in the New Age's attitude to wealth and work, far-reaching changes have occurred in the nature of the work with which New Agers have been involved. Working life in contemporary Western societies demands an evr-increasing degree of ontological flexibility. Personality is quickly becoming a raw material for commercial exploitation by employers (McDonald 1993). New Age self-transformative practices are tools with which people can remake themselves much more readily while attaching some greater meaning to this loss of a stable sense of self and loss of a predictable social environment, and thereby enable some people to thrive in the ontological turbulence surrounding postmodern flexibility (Ziguras 1997b). Richards describes the role of New Age ideologies in encouraging workers to be autonomous, self-steering and entrepreneurial in the face of the dismantling of corporate structures which are claimed to have encouraged dependency (see Roberts 1994). As management adopts models of organizational control which emphasize the devolution of power and enhanced reflexivity on the part of individuals and groups within the organization, there is a need to change the 'culture' of the workplace either by retrenching and re-hiring on a casual basis or through personality and behavioural modification of existing workers. In this latter project of instilling desired motivations in a workforce, the New Age has been very successful in selling its services to corporations, governments and the self-employed. Contemporary management training has embraced New Age notions of self-empowerment and self-transformation in order to mould their workers' desires to conform with the organizational requirement for flexibility (Roberts 1994). The New Age's celebration of constant change as in itself meaningful and its recasting of perpetual psychological upheaval as the essence of the 'spiritual journey' is put to corporate use in allaying the anxieties which stem from decreasing job security.

Advertising and the detraditionalization of self-care

The production and consumption of self-care have now been comprehensively incorporated into the market, and the informal reproduction of self-care practices has been overwhelmed by the commercial production and promotion of commodified self-care advice, techniques and tools. Thus commercial self-care promotion has an interest in heightening the consumer's sense of behavioural autonomy, promoting a sense of personal responsibility for health and overemphasizing their ability to influence their health. Michael Parenti describes the cumulative impact these messages have on audiences:

> The reader of advertising copy and the viewer of commercials discover that they are not doing right for baby's needs or hubby's or wifey's desires; that they are failing in their careers because of poor appearance, sloppy dress; that they are not treating their complexion, hair or nails properly; that they

suffer unnecessary cold misery and headache pains; that they do not know how to make the tastiest coffee, pie, pudding or chicken dinner; nor, if left to their own devices, would they be able to clean their floors, sinks and toilets correctly or tend to their own lawns, gardens, appliances, and automobiles. In order to live well and live properly, consumers need corporate producers to guide them. Consumers are taught personal incompetence and dependence on mass-market producers.

(Parenti 1986: 65)

While undermining cultural traditions of self-care, making individuals more vulnerable to uncertainty and health-related anxiety, capitalism sells the promise of ontological security back to consumers. Strictly speaking, reflexive self-care practices themselves cannot be fully commodified as they are both produced and consumed by the same person; however, everything surrounding them has been absorbed into the market: advice and instructions on how to care for one's self; information about health risks to assist decision-making; tools and equipment to be used on the self; and medications and health foods to be consumed. For simplicity's sake, however, I will still refer to entry of all these associated practices into the market as the commodification of self-care.

In the industrial phase of capitalism, the development of new means of production radically transformed the world in which people lived. Marx and other nineteenth-century social theorists were in awe of capitalism's ability to cause cultural change on a scale never before known, uprooting traditional ways of life and replacing them with more temporary and more fluid circumstances, and the dynamism of the capitalist mode of production has continued to transform conditions of life to this day (Berman 1982). At the same time, the increasing commodification of culture made possible by the advent of various mass media has heightened the power of market in the shaping of self-identity. The history of self-help books provides an example of this process in which informal cultural reproduction became overlaid by the commercial production of culture in mediated form.

Until the late nineteenth century, advertising had been produced by local or regional entrepreneurs in trade cards, calendars and almanacs. The emergence of integrated national markets, broader circulation print media and larger corporations brought with them a new form of advertising which communicated brand names to national markets. These new agencies continued a tradition of associating products with claims of physical and psychic revitalization, a strategy that had a long history in the evangelical culture of nineteenth-century America. Their products' magical cures and amazing self-transformations closely resembled contemporary descriptions of religious awakening. Already in nineteenth-century health advertising, the model of health employed in advertising was more vital and energetic than earlier popular conceptions. Each product tried to outdo its competitors in terms of the beneficial effects that it claimed to possess. It was not enough to claim to relieve specific symptoms when other products were claiming to do this plus increase the consumer's vitality, increase their performance and improve their whole outlook on life (Lears 1989).

The new advertising agencies also introduced Enlightenment themes into commercial promotions. Leaders of the advertising industry at the end of the nineteenth century claimed to be spearheading a major cultural transformation. In 1909 one New York-based advertising agency asserted that

> advertising is *revolutionary*. Its tendency is to overturn preconceived notions, to set new ideas spinning through the reader's brain, to induce something that they never did before. It is a form of progress, and it *interests only progressive people*. That's why it thrives in America as in no other land under the sun. Stupid people are not much impressed by advertising. They move in the rut of tradition.
>
> (cited in Lears 1989: 49)

Larger audience-reach and larger budgets gave these new cultural producers a sense of their power to transform social life on a historic scale. The shift from local to national markets allowed for the unprecedented rationalization and standardization of cultural life. In traditional societies, self-care practices were relatively local because people were able to experience only what they could encounter first-hand. Stories carried by travellers about distant events were generally sketchy and unreliable, while knowledge about the shared locales of everyday life was built up over generations, constantly reiterated and re-experienced. One would expect that in recent years Madison Avenue advertising executives would be similarly conscious of a new phase of the expansion of their cultural power facilitated by the rapid globalization of national media and markets.

The rise of the metropolitan agencies also saw a shift from romantic to scientistic claims in health advertising around the turn of the twentieth century. In the nineteenth century, American advertisements for self-care products were steeped in a herbalist lore which emphasized the product's closeness to nature and magical effects. The national advertisers appealed more routinely to scientific claims and relied more heavily on images of youthful physical perfection. Lears notes that in the United States, the 'voluptuous woman and the bearded man yielded to smoother, cleaner, more activist and athletic models of beauty' (Lears 1989: 56). The iconography of the body became more sterilized and controlled with the corporatization of advertising. In part this was a reflection of the culture of the advertising agencies themselves, which were metropolitan and highly educated. On a broader scale, however, this shift reflected the contemporary preoccupations of an urban middle class who sought to make their homes as sanitary or sterile as possible. The popularization of germ theory had combined with the age-old tendency for upper classes to seek to distinguish themselves from lower classes by contrasting their 'cultured' lifestyles with the 'natural' conditions of the toiling masses. Cleanliness and physical fitness thus became central features in the reassertion of bourgeois superiority. 'It was no accident', Lears observes, 'that the ideal males in advertisements began to look like heroes from that burgeoning realm of upper-class revitalization, the college football field, or that ideal females looked like their co-ed admirers' (Lears 1989: 61). This elevation of the urban middle-class body aesthetic through a powerful advertising industry established the hegemonic middle-class standard of physical perfection which has since become firmly entrenched.

After the Second World War, the advertising industry began to use new techniques to tap into consumers' unconscious and subconscious motivations rather than simply appealing to them as rational agents (Packard 1957). Advertisers and marketers in the fifties became increasingly aware of the pitfalls of treating their audiences as rational consumers, after it became clear that consumers would often not tell market researchers the truth about what they wanted. There was a new emphasis on how people felt about products rather than what they thought about them. Because of the relatively impersonal nature of the disembodied modes of communication when compared with face-to-face interaction, those who produce mediated communications must constantly struggle to create an emotional impact in audiences. This emotional distance also allows producers to transcend limits imposed on face-to-face interactions. Semi-naked bodies are displayed much more readily on television than in real life, where the gratuitous display of flesh would be considered inappropriate. Likewise public health advertisements regularly use shocking images and scenarios in order to scare their audiences into an emotional response which will heighten their recall of the message in key situations and cause people to talk to others about the advertisement and hence the message, and hence reinforce this message interpersonally. Nevertheless, there is an ongoing debate as to the effectiveness of such shock tactics (Australian Medical Association 1997, Brow 1997).

Featherstone (1987) points out that the instrumental and expressive qualities of commodities can no longer be treated as separate because so much of the use value of commodities in consumer culture is in the image the product expresses. The market has thus increased its reach into the shaping of identity and the production of cultural life through adding expressive value to commodities. The commodification of personal identity has in this way now expanded historically to encompass all aspects of self-identity, including appearance, sexuality, demeanour and self-care. Contemporary lifestyles are conglomerations of commodified objects and practices which are fashioned together by a consumer who experiences the creation of their lifestyle as the active self-expression of their own individual identity. Within the resulting consumer culture, the individual is constantly reminded by advertising that not only their clothes, but every one of their possessions – their home, car, CD collection, haircut – as well as every one of their non-material consumption choices will be judged according to hierarchies of taste. In such a culture, the cultural meanings of self-care practices are increasingly shaped through advertising and the commercial provision of lifestyle advice.

This new phase of commodification of culture and self-identity has been integrally related to the development of new means of mass communication, which allowed for the dramatic expansion of the dissemination of information and images. For example, the aestheticization of mass production and the rise of the fashion industry went hand in hand with the development of photography, which allowed for a dramatic increase in the communication of the expressive qualities of goods through pictorial advertising. Similarly, the commercial promotion of self-care advice in its current form has been made possible by the advent of television, magazines, video, radio, and so on.

Since the late twentieth century, one of the dominant themes of health-related advertising industry has been to emphasize the individual's freedom to manage their own health. Even smoking advertisements appeal to consumers to exercise their autonomy by using their products. In 1995, Rothmans, one of Australia's three tobacco companies, ran an advertising campaign aimed at drawing attention to the limitations on the rights of smokers. Rothmans hired political lobbyist Richard Farmer to orchestrate a smokers' rights campaign which involved billboard advertisements in Australian capital cities which simply read 'Personal Liberty is the Right of Every Australian'. A recent amendment to tobacco advertising laws had allowed tobacco companies their constitutional right to freedom of political speech to communicate 'solely on political and government matters' after a High Court challenge to the legislation by the tobacco industry. The ads were legal as long as they carried no mention of cigarettes or anything identifying them as Rothmans' promotions. Farmer spoke to reporters extensively as the advertisements were launched so that the news media carried the message that these were pro-smoking statements, which the ads themselves could not state. Rothmans had earlier released a new brand of cigarettes onto the Australian market called Freedom. They carried a quote from Abraham Lincoln on the side of the packet: 'Those who deny freedom to others deserve it not for themselves' (Haigh 1995). Rothmans sought to arouse resentment against the restrictions placed upon the tobacco industry and the restrictions on smoking in workplaces and many enclosed public spaces. This served a dual purpose. It obviously endeavoured to put pressure on health authorities further to justify their restrictions on market 'freedom'. A more subtle, but more powerful, intention, however, was to cultivate in smokers a sense of free-spirited rebelliousness, which would provide them with the rhetoric with which to mount a respectable defence of their right to degrade their own health. This attempt to encourage smokers to express their individuality by smoking is made explicit in statements to the press at the time the posters were launched. Announcing its campaign launch, Rothmans quoted 'the voice of ordinary Australian smokers' as saying:

> I don't think adults should be telling other adults what to do. We all know the risks and we smoke because that is our choice. We don't need someone telling us what is wrong and what harm we are doing to ourselves. [...] I think the anti-smokers' push – I don't really believe they are so interested in

your health. It's more of a social engineering thing, bit of a power trip really.

(cited in R. Campbell 1995)

The language of rights is employed effectively here in terms of a right to harm oneself. While the company described the campaign as an attempt to change attitudes to *smokers* both on a cultural and political level, through such statements they were obviously attempting to change attitudes to *smoking*. Smoking is cast as an assertion of non-conformism. Coinciding with the launch, Rothmans released the results of an ANOP (Australian National Opinion Polls) poll they had commissioned which they said showed that 65 per cent of adult smokers believed that governments, pressure groups and employers were too involved in restricting personal rights (R. Campbell 1995). Farmer told readers of Brisbane's *Courier Mail* that 'the state has no right telling the people what they can and can't do with their own body' (cited in Swanwick 1995). He urged readers of the *Adelaide Advertiser* to fight back, arguing that 'smokers are fed up with the intolerance being preached by the anti-smoking movement. [...] The petty minded non-smoking people have turned SA [South Australia] into a nanny State' (Read 1995). Similar articles covering Farmer's smokers' rights argument appeared in all major daily newspapers in the country, and even though Rothmans must have known that much of the reporting of their campaign would be critical, their message got through to smokers and potential smokers through Farmer's rhetoric nonetheless (McKimmie 1995).

Advertising necessarily constructs the consumer's actions as free choice at the same time as it seeks to shape their actions in a certain direction. This is most visible in the tobacco industry's defence of its 'right' to advertise. The tobacco industry, of course, argues that advertising does not encourage people to smoke. If this were the case, however, it would be the only product for which advertising was not able to affect levels of consumption. In the words of a former president and chairman of the board of the world's second largest advertising agency:

> In recent years the cigarette industry has been artfully maintaining that cigarette advertising has nothing to do with total sales. [...] I am always amused by the suggestion that advertising, a function which has been shown to increase consumption with virtually every other product, somehow mirac- ulously fails to work for tobacco products. The industry only advances this argument to try to undermine efforts to restrict tobacco promotion.
>
> (cited in Anti-Cancer Council of Victoria 1990: 7)

While this may be right, there may be another reason for the tobacco industry claims that advertising does not induce people to smoke. The message is also aimed at smokers, who need to be assured that they are not being 'duped' into smoking by advertising but are choosing 'freely'. This is an issue not only in tobacco advertising but also in all forms of advertising in which the consumption of a product is constitutive of the consumer's sense of autonomy. Advertisers never overtly instruct people how to act, but rather ask them to choose a certain product.

By contrast with this 'empowering' approach, public health promotion communications quite often instruct the audience in the 'correct' way of behaving. This is not without its difficulties. Consider, for example, the problems faced by health-care institutions who seek to engage in public health education through the mass media. In using the media to change self-care practices, the state seems relatively powerless in the face of the vastly greater levels of commercial advertising spending. As health promotion organizations are the first to admit, using the mass media to convey 'official' health information often proves difficult for other reasons as well. The (American) National Cancer Institute's guide for health promoters, *Making Health Communications Work*, begins with a typically pessimistic preface:

> Communicating effectively about health is a difficult task. Health information is often complex and technical. In addition, the information may be inconclusive, controversial, contradictory, and subject to change as new research findings are released. Many diseases such as cancer are fear arousing; individual responses may be emotional. New health information may conflict with long-held personal beliefs. As a result, the potential exists for misdirecting or alienating the public.
>
> (National Cancer Institute 1997)

Health promotion agencies seek to use the mass media to achieve much more profound behavioural change than the purchase of a specific product. Where governments have used the mass media in an intensive way for proactive self-care promotion, it is usually as part of a broad campaign incorporating advertisements, press-releases, education of professionals, legislative action and school-based education. The Australian anti-skin cancer campaign provides a good example of the use of the mass media in such a way. Early detection campaigns commenced in the 1960s with the expansion of melanoma screening but it was not until the 1981 'Slip! Slop! Slap!' advertising campaign that a national strategy of television, radio and magazine advertisements sought to change behavioural patterns that increase the risk of skin cancer. This was accompanied by efforts in schools and sporting groups to require sun-protection wear to be worn by children in organized settings. Each year at the beginning of summer the National Skin Cancer Awareness Week introduces a new theme to supplement the accrued messages. By the mid-1990s, health workers could state that the messages had 'reached into almost every aspect of daily life in Australia' due to the combined effects of public health campaigns, school-based education and the commercial promotion of products such as shade screens, sunglasses and sun-screen (Marks 1994). Similarly, anti-smoking videos and print information have been shown to be much more effective when they are supplemented with participation in self-help groups (Jason *et al.* 1995). For public health interventions, which aim at lasting and significant behavioural change, disembodied communication is generally more effective if accompanied by interaction with professionals and face-to-face care.

With commodification, social practices which were once taken-for-granted and rooted in reciprocal relationships are transformed into choices which the individual must make on a more conscious level. The necessity to choose between a plethora of options makes us aware of our own capacity to choose, making us feel self-constitutive. With the commodification of lifestyle, the individual consumer has the experience of being able actively to create their own identity. The market celebrates the freedom of choice that the consumer is faced with and, however minimal that choice may appear to distant observers, the consumer experiences the restrictions on their ability to choose as limitations emanating from outside the market – the faltering economy, their own inability to earn more spending money, or government interference. This sense of being able actively to create one's self and one's life is partially an outcome of the necessity to engage in discriminating choice. People want to believe that the choices which they make are made freely, within the obvious monetary constraints. As we will see in the next section, however, advertising works by continually affirming the consumer's freedom in the market in order to hide the power which works through its own rhetoric.

The perception that one's lifestyle and expressed identity can be freely chosen raises major crises of authenticity, or identity crises, in which the person is faced with the realization that they may not 'really' be the person they have made themselves into. Alvin Toffler has discussed the ontological consequences of what he calls 'overchoice':

> The intensification of the problem of overchoice presses us towards orgies of self-examination, soul-searching and introversion. It confronts us with that most popular of contemporary illnesses, the 'identity crisis'. [...] Each time we make a style choice, a super-decision, each time we link up with some particular subcultural group or groups, we make some change in our self-image. We become, in some sense, a different person, and we perceive ourselves as different. Our old friends, those who knew us in some previous incarnation, raise their eyebrows. They have a harder and harder time recognizing us, and, in fact, we experience increasing difficulty in identifying with, or even sympathizing with, our own past selves.
>
> (Toffler 1971: 289–90)

Some of these choices subsequently become routinized as habits which allow the person some continuity of identity and the possibility of avoiding constantly making decisions. This is necessary for establishing a basic level of ontological security. There is a strong potential in such an apparently open field of 'self-constitution' for the dissolution of a stable and whole sense of identity, and the loss of ontological security. It is worth elaborating what ontological security means in this context. In R.D. Laing's description,

> a basically ontologically secure person will encounter all the hazards of life, social, ethical, spiritual, biological, from a centrally firm sense of his [*sic*] own and other people's reality and identity. [...] they have a sense of their integral selfhood and personal identity, of the permanency of things, of the reliability of natural processes, of the substantiality of others.
>
> (Laing 1965: 39)

The identity crises which result from ontological insecurity include such symptoms as confusion about values, feelings of vagueness and emptiness, detachment from and loss of interest in everyday life, generalized anxiety, self-consciousness and an over-examined life, confusion, bewilderment and discouragement (Sharp 1985).

The market has been able to exploit the existential problems of the consumer society, not only providing the materials with which consumers can construct their identity, but also providing as part of the package confirmation of the worth of the self which is being projected. This is a constant process of undermining and shoring up identity through consumption. Marketing actively undermines existing integrative practices and existing ontological security in order to change consumers' behaviour to adopt a new product. When marketers battle with each other to affirm or undermine a consumer's self-worth, they are only concerned with having that consumer's self-worth attached to their product. This perpetual affirming and undermining of the consumer's self-worth and ontological security fuels demand for new and better products which will satisfy their insecurities. The increase in the emotionality of consumption draws the consumer into this cycle of dependence in ways which progress ever deeper into the psyche of the person (Hochschild 1983).

In the space of a few generations, the intense and rapid commodification of self-care has altered dramatically the way in which it is produced and consumed, with individual practices now heavily influenced by commercial cultural production. There are close parallels between the expropriation of self-care and the expropriation of popular music, the telling of stories, the making of clothes, or any other aspect of the production of culture. Popular music became commodified once the writing and performance of popular songs was taken over by professional singers and musicians, rather than being composed and performed in a less 'orchestrated' way on a smaller scale by 'the people themselves'. With the medicalization of life, self-care is expropriated, commodified and reconstructed through the professional-institutional level of integration. A major motivating factor for the carer is the income they receive for providing assistance, which is potentially in conflict with the interests of the patient. As a result, a key feature of the process of professionalization was the development of professional ethics which regulated the potentially competing interests of the provider and consumer of care. It is interesting to note that one major criticism of the alternative therapies is that they lack such institutional regulation and codes of ethics which would prevent practitioners from providing fee-paying patients with popular, but largely ineffective, therapies motivated by profit rather than the health of their patients (for example, see Maddocks 1985; Coward 1989; Furnham 1994). Now, in an age of deregulation, the professional power of medicine is coming under further threat in the name of consumer empowerment. In Australia the push to introduce competition in the health sector has led to an end to the prohibition of medical advertising, which has long been enforced by medical boards (Lyall 1997). In the United States, a ban on advertising prescription drugs to the general public was lifted in 1997, and soon after, Eli Lilly, the manufacturers of Prozac, ran advertisements offering university scholarships to schizophrenic patients who switched to their latest anti-psychotic medication (Josefson 1998). This type of 'freeing up' of the health-care market has had the effect of undermining the authority of individual medical practitioners by encouraging consumers to shop-around while at the same time increasing the power of large medical chains and pharmaceutical corporations which are able to attract consumers through the mass media.

Health advice online

Most people who use the Internet, the surveys tell us, have at one time or another searched for the answers to their own health problems. If you have ever done this, you will know that there are hundreds of pages of information on even the most obscure conditions. Consequently, doctors now encounter an increasing number of patients who have already researched their condition on the Web. They come into the clinic armed with print-outs containing lists of side-effects written by the wary, advertisements written by the producers, warnings written by the unsatisfied, and page after page of 'balanced' advice written by a host of authorities of varying reputation.

In the last year or two the health-care sector has begun to take the Internet seriously. Pharmaceutical companies are now using the Web to appeal directly to consumers, commercial health information sites with substantial corporate backing are springing up, and governments are finally beginning to produce public health information sites of their own.

But what are the effects of this proliferation of health information on the Web? The most common claim is that the Web is democratizing health information and empowering health-care consumers in relation to providers (Hardey 1999). If you walk into a doctor's surgery or a pharmacy with a bundle of print-outs in your hand, you and the person in the white coat are on a more level playing field. The Web facilitates self-medication, allowing patients to be more active in their own diagnosis and treatment. These empowered patients use professionals as consultants and tend to shop around more. While other electronic media are good at 'pushing' information at broad audiences, the World Wide Web is much better at providing more targeted information which can be 'pulled' by individual users on demand. Empowered consumers can do their own homework on the Web, and there is growing demand by patients to be able to e-mail queries to health-care professionals and receive advice and prescriptions over the wires. Needless to say, most doctors are less than excited about this possibility.

Neo-liberals celebrate this patient empowerment through the Internet, and their most visible spokesperson is perhaps Dr C. Everett Koop, who was US Surgeon General during the Reagan years. He used his public image to help form one of the most popular health sites on the Web, Dr Koop.com (*www.drkoop.com*). The site, Koop claims, 'empowers consumers to become active, well-informed participants to better manage their health'. The site was launched in 1998 with its stated focus to 'change healthcare in America by empowering individuals with the information and resources they need to take charge of their own health'. By 1999, Drkoop.com had over one million registered users and its revenue is growing exponentially, allowing it to build a network of alliances with other leading health and wellness e-commerce sites, including a US$30 million deal with Selfcare.com (*www.selfcare.com*).

In one way, Koop is right in observing that the prevalence of health information on the Web 'is going to change the whole paradigm we've been used to in medicine' (Davis and Miller 1999). It may slowly change the relationship between some patients and doctors, but this has already been happening for a long time. The amount of health advice in the mass media has increased dramatically in recent decades, corresponding to dramatic changes in the way self-care advice is produced and communicated. In the 1960s and early 1970s the power of the medical profession was at its peak and social critics were becoming increasingly concerned at the medicalization of everyday life. However, the profession was already beginning to lose its hold over the population as advertising, self-help books and various other sources of commercial and public health information provided patients with second and third opinions before they had even stepped into the clinic.

At the same time, governments around the world began encouraging individuals to take responsibility for themselves as a means of preventing illness and reducing health care costs. The Reagan government (with Koop as Surgeon General) embraced their own version of 'self-help', a term which had previously been the political preserve of Left liberals. Reagan was happy to dismantle public institutions, scrap social welfare provisions and let the mentally ill care for themselves on the streets of America. The New Right spoke of 'restrictive' services being replaced with the 'free flow' of information, thereby providing consumers with freedom of choice (Turem and Born 1983).

This rationale was employed throughout the economically developed countries by conservative governments that sought to cut public health services. During the 1990s, the head of the Victorian Department of Human Services in Australia who oversaw dramatic cuts to the public health system argued that the introduction of market mechanisms in health care was finally possible because new information technologies would allow consumers to overcome the power of health-care providers. Health-care systems would only operate efficiently, he argued, once the political distortions in the system were eliminated. This could be achieved, he proposed, by using information technology 'to provide the consumer with information, and from that, choice and control. We are accustomed to being in control of most aspects of our lives. It is time health care caught up' (Paterson 1966:1). For example, he suggested increasing the supply of information about the effectiveness of various treatment options so that consumers could make more autonomous choices about their care.

Given the often superficial and unreliable nature of much health information, health-care professionals are understandably concerned at such suggestions (McClung *et al.* 1998). While market fundamentalists argue that diagnostic and therapeutic decisions can be made by individuals with access to the Internet, then seek out the practitioner and treatment option of their choice, less anti-medical commentators paint a picture of mediated information, professionals and patients all working together towards the same end. According to Koop, 'Patients are getting more and more control because of the knowledge they have [...] which enables them to make decisions *with* their doctor about diagnosis, procedures and treatment' (quoted in Davis and Miller 1999, emphasis added).

One flaw in the empowerment thesis is the enormous variety of sources of health advice on the Web and the lack of any regulation of content quality compared with other media. The trouble is that the Internet is not simply a large medical textbook, and people who study online information aren't necessarily going to come to the same conclusions as their health-care practitioners. To illustrate the preponderance of non-scientifically based information on the Web, a group of researchers at the University of Sydney with a long-standing interest in the anti-immunization movement used seven leading search engines to locate information on the search terms 'immunization' (with an 's' or a 'z') and 'vaccination'. Close to half of the top ten search results were anti-immunization sites, and on Google, all of the first ten results opposed vaccination. The researchers noted that the sites sometimes had scientific-sounding names and often used scientific language to dress up anecdotes as reliable research (Swan 2002).

In response, articles helping Web surfers to interpret the masses of health information on the Web now appear regularly in magazines, newspapers and on television lifestyle programmes. These usually aim to help readers evaluate the authenticity of health sites by directing their attention to the publishing organization, authors' affiliations and credentials, attribution of sources of information, disclosure of ownership of site, advertising and sponsorship details, and currency of information.

Developing Web users' ability to discern 'quality' information addresses the demand side of the online health information issue, and on the supply side several organizations have developed codes of conduct to try to improve the quality of the information that appears on the Web. Such codes have not yet made significant impact on the supply of various types of information, and at this point, while there is a level of agreement among health-care practitioners about which institutions and which sites they should trust, the public has a much more difficult time assessing 'quality' health advice online. The most ambitious of these efforts was a proposal by the World Health Organization (WHO) to establish a 'dot health' domain name for the Internet, allowing the WHO to authorize and thereby provide quality assurance for sites using the .health extension. This plan was rejected in 2000 by the authority that oversees top-level domain names on the Internet, the Internet Corporation for Assigned Names and Numbers (ICANN), who were anxious about such forms of content control. More recently, the European Commission in 2002 adopted a set of six Quality Criteria for Health-Related Websites: transparency and honesty; authority; privacy and data protection; updating of information; accountability; and accessibility. These quality criteria will inform future action by Member States, national and regional health authorities and content producers and may be implemented through more detailed codes of conduct, self-applied codes or quality labels, user guidance tools, filtering tools, third-party quality and accreditation systems, and possibly a system of recognizable EU seals of approval for Internet sites (European Commission 2002).

Even if such quality assurance ventures succeed, there will still be considerable diversity of advice from sites deemed to be acceptable. To test the accuracy of medically respectable sites, a research team in 1997 surveyed sixty websites sponsored by physicians, nurses and university medical centres, comparing the advice they provided on treating childhood diarrhoea with the recommendations of the American Academy of Pediatrics. Eighty per cent of these sites contained inaccurate information, and academic institutions' websites were no more accurate than sources devoted to alternative therapies such as herbalism and chiropractic (Kiernan 1998).

Government sites are often static and dull, and tend to be repositories of impersonal facts about diseases written in overly technical and bureaucratic language. By comparison, the large commerical sites such as iVillage, Selfcare.com and Dr Koop.com, resemble online magazines, but with the addition of encyclopedic resource databases, interactive discussion areas and online health product stores. Two of the largest sites, WebMD and Medscape (*www.medscape.com*), have both a professional-oriented site and a consumer/patient-oriented site with different formats, content and styles. Advertising revenue and capital investment allow large commercial sites to provide comprehensive, well-written, regularly updated information. As early as 1999, Glaxo Wellcome paid the women's health website iVillage (*www.ivillage.com*) over US$1.7 million for a one-year sponsorship deal (Davis and Miller 1999). Nevertheless, despite this advertising revenue (most commonly for pharmaceuticals), which generates most of the income for the large commercial sites, they remain unprofitable, like many other Web commerce ventures (Newman 2001).

While all the sites discussed so far aim to distribute information from experts to lay audiences, perhaps the most significant use of the Internet is to connect people with similar health issues. There are numerous online chat rooms, mailing lists and websites created by community-based organizations dedicated to every conceivable condition, and a newly diagnosed sufferer can often find a community of people ready to share their own experiences and offer support. The dissemination of information 'horizontally', between community-based groups on the Web, provides a diversity of resources, in contrast to the medical dominance of most 'top-down' official sites. A British study recently found that nearly three-quarters of self-help groups and voluntary organizations in the field of neurology had a Web presence, and all of the groups that did not were planning to do so in the future (N. Fox 2001).

Part of the reason government and community groups have been slow onto the Internet is that the people who have access to the Net are generally from the healthiest part of the population. The three 'C's, as the American's call them – cash, college and computers – go hand in hand, and those on the wired side of the digital divide live longer and are healthier than the unwired part of the population. Any resources devoted to improving the health of the online population may simply increase this inequality in health status.

As the Internet becomes increasingly commercialized, it is likely that it will go the way of television. Nobody these days would argue that the major effect of television on the health of populations has been to increase the flow of information thereby leading to healthier lifestyles. Product advertising has had a far greater impact on lifestyle change than health promotion campaigns or the dissemination of expert knowledge. A New Zealand study of food ads targeted at children explains the consequences of the types of behavioural changes that food advertising promotes:

> Children who ate only the advertised foods would eat a diet too high in fat, saturated fat, protein, free sugars and sodium. [...] The food products advertised [...] rarely included nutritious low-cost foods that are necessary for food security in low-income groups. There were also no food advertisements that included any of the healthy foods consumed by Maori and Pacific peoples.
>
> (Wilson *et al.* 1999: 247)

The same will likely occur online – there is no rush to sell fruit and vegetables online but every commercial health site is selling vitamin pills. The second similar health effect of television worth noting is that it causes physical inactivity. The American Academy of Pediatrics has warned that 'increased television use is documented to be a significant factor leading to obesity' (American Academy of Pediatrics 1999: 341). American researchers have found that they could cause children to lose weight simply by reducing the number of hours of TV they watch (Robinson 1999). How long will it be before a medical research team shows that you can improve a person's level of physical health and sense of well-being by hiding their mouse for a couple of weeks?

4 Natural alternatives

When conditions of life for any animal population deviate from those to which it is genetically adapted, biological maladjustment – discordance – is inevitable. The human species is no exception. For us, the discordance between our current lifestyle and the one in which in which we evolved has promoted the chronic and deadly 'diseases of civilization': the heart attacks, strokes, cancer, diabetes, emphysema, hypertension, cirrhosis, and like illnesses that cause 75 per cent of all mortality in the United States and other industrialized nations.

S. Boyd Eaton, Majorie Shostak and Melvin Konner, *The Paleolithic Prescription* (1988: 5)

If civilization is the disease, 'natural' self-care is the cure. The range of therapeutic systems labelled 'alternative' or 'complementary' differ from each other in many ways, but share a faith in the capacity for preventive self-care and reactive 'self-healing' by living in harmony with embodied nature. The best-known of these are acupuncture, aromatherapy, herbal medicine, hypnosis, massage and yoga (Furnham 2000). Alternative practitioners and patients are more likely to see the practitioner as a consultant in their own self-care, and likewise practitioners place more emphasis on the person as an active agent in their own care. Since the early 1970s there has been a dramatic increase in the popular use and acceptance of alternative therapies in contemporary Western societies. In these relatively new therapeutic systems, the interaction between practitioner and patient is more thoroughly framed by the disembodied level of social integration. The professional-institutional authority of the practitioner is deliberately played down, and instead a large proportion of their authority derives from the correspondence between the practitioner's beliefs and that of the patient, both of whom are informed by a natural therapeutic culture communicated through disembodied means. That is, alternative medicine is much more integrated into a culture of proactive self-care, relying on the patient's access to and familiarity with many sources of disembodied advice. Orthodox medical practice, by contrast, has been relatively slow to respond to this proliferation of self-care advice in the print and electronic media.

Given the very different genealogies and contemporary practices of the health-care systems which are lumped under these terms, what basis is there for speaking of 'alternative medicine' in the singular rather than 'alternative

medicines' in the plural? This objection is often made by advocates of a particular alternative therapy who resent being tarred with the same brush as other
alternative therapies they consider radically different or highly dubious. The
alternative modalities do exhibit vast differences in their historical development,
their methods of diagnosis, their treatments, their legitimacy within the mainstream health-care system, their efficacy, their popularity, and so on, but for the
purposes of my argument here there is considerable consistency between them.
Despite these differences, which I in no way want to deny, it is possible to identify
a number of common themes within alternative medicine. While the content of
their practices and discourses varies widely, at a more abstract level they share
common features which serve to structure their content in similar ways.

Most of these therapies were developed outside orthodox health-care systems
and were often the object of distrust, if not open antagonism. Many define
'alternative medicine' as 'those branches of the art and science of health care
that are not in accordance with current medical thought, scientific knowledge or
university teaching' (Ernst 1994: 121). The term 'alternative medicine' has been
dropped by many advocates of these therapies, for two main reasons. Firstly,
more positive descriptions which emphasize commonalities rather than their
shared exclusion are preferred by most advocates, typically terms such as
'natural therapies', 'holistic health care', and so on. The term 'complementary' is
now preferred by many groups on both sides of the divide to emphasize the
compatibility of these therapeutic systems with orthodox medicine (British
Medical Association 1993). Governments have also generally been opposed to
the promotion of any system of treatment as an alternative to orthodox
medicine and for that reason have preferred names which emphasize compatibility and co-existence rather than opposition (O'Neill 1994: 53–4).

Opposition by orthodox medicine has excluded many new therapies from the
mainstream health-care system and attempts by medical authorities strictly to
demarcate orthodoxy have resulted in a dichotomization of therapeutic systems.
Orthodox medical practitioners have claimed the right to protect the public from
the harm which they believe non-biomedical health-care practitioners may
cause. Although this oppositional stance has softened in recent years, they often
brand alternative practitioners as unscientific quacks who are either deluding
themselves or knowingly exploiting public ignorance (Gevitz 1988). The medical
profession commonly refers to alternative medicine in more polite terms as
'placebo medicine', seeing its popularity and value stemming only from the more
personal relationships established between patient and practitioner and the use
of more pleasant and uplifting therapies (Maddocks 1985).

Up until the twentieth century there was little that orthodox medicine could
do to stop what it saw as 'fringe' health-care practitioners. As orthodox medicine
obtained state patronage in the late nineteenth and early twentieth centuries,
coupled with considerable success in the treatment of transmissible diseases,
many other therapeutic systems were increasingly marginalized and restricted.
The more traditional forms of healing, handed down from one practitioner to
their successor through an apprenticeship system of hands-on training (as was

generally the way for medical education until the twentieth century), were predominantly the preserve of women. When orthodox medicine, the preserve of upper-class men, obtained state patronage and subsidization for its institutions, it was able to extend its reach into the general population. Alternative therapies had no access to state research and educational institutions and were actively discredited and subject to a range of legal sanctions which restricted the provision of non-medical health care (Willis 1989).

In recent decades, however, the popularity of alternative therapies has increased dramatically. Studies in the United States and Australia generally estimate that between 10 per cent and 20 per cent of these populations consult unconventional practitioners each year. Eisenberg *et al.* (1993) famously found that 12 per cent of respondents visited unconventional practitioners, with that group averaging nineteen visits per year. When these figures were extrapolated to the US population as a whole, they suggest that Americans made 425 million visits to providers of non-conventional therapies, which is more than the total number of consultations with orthodox primary-care physicians, estimated at 388 million. Expenditures related to this use of non-conventional practitioners is estimated at US$13.7 billion, three-quarters of which was paid for out-of-pocket, which is comparable to the US$12.8 billion spent out-of-pocket annually for hospitalization in the United States. Around the same time, an Australian study found that nearly half of the children with cancer they surveyed had used at least one alternative therapy, without the child's doctors' knowledge in most cases (Sawyer *et al.* 1994). A 1996 study estimated that Australian consumers spent A$621 million each year on alternative medicines (far greater than the A$360 million of patient contributions to all pharmaceutical drugs purchased in Australia at that time) with a further A$309 million spent on alternative practitioners each year (MacLennan *et al.* 1996). By the end of the decade, alternative and complementary therapies were so accepted in the United States that the National Centre for Complementary and Alternative Therapies budget had risen to US$100 million per year and two-thirds of US medical colleges offered courses in these previously marginalized therapeutics (Cowley 2002).

Why are people seeking out alternative therapies? Three major factors help to explain the dramatic increase in the popularity of alternative medicine since the 1970s: firstly, a disillusionment concerning the efficacy of orthodox medicine; secondly, a preference for a less authoritarian and more 'empowering' patient–practitioner relationship; and thirdly, a preference for 'natural' therapeutic and self-care techniques.

Efficacy

In studies of attitudinal differences between users of alternative medicine and the general population, one recurrent theme is a scepticism about the claimed efficacy of orthodox medicine (Sheehan 1984; Furnham and Smith 1988). Doctors like to think that alternative therapies are a last resort for those whom orthodox medicine cannot help, and that the popularity of alternative therapies rises and falls historically depending on orthodox medicine's ability to provide acceptable treatments to the major health problems of the day (Holden 1978). In many cases this is true, but users of alternative therapies are also acting out of dissatisfaction with their medical care and a preference for safe natural methods (Victorian Government Social Development Committee 1986).

Alternative therapies are generally used alongside orthodox medical services. In Canada, a study of the health behaviour of chiropractic patients found that they did not use any fewer prescription medicines than did the population as a whole; however, they were more likely to use other alternative therapies and took more non-prescription medicines (Northcott and Bachynsky 1993). Elderly users of chiropractic are also more likely to be users of physician services than are non-chiropractic patients (Shapiro 1983). There is some evidence to suggest that users of alternative medicine also make more use of orthodox services.

Alternative therapies are used more by patients with chronic and non-life-threatening conditions, primarily musculo-skeletal complaints and minor ailments such as headaches and sinus problems (Eisenberg *et al.* 1993). Alternative medicine tends to treat predominantly those conditions which orthodox medicine is less successful in treating. This preference for treating chronic conditions contrasts sharply with orthodox medicine's record, which has shown considerable advances in the treatment of acute disease and trauma, but significantly less publicly acclaimed inroads into the care of the less critically ill. Acute illness is taken to be the end result of considerable and lengthy unwellness, so that alternative therapies, which aim to assist the body's preventive mechanisms, have little to offer at this stage. Nor is alternative medicine particularly good at treating epidemic diseases and injury, but it can have an adjunct role in assisting recuperation. These therapies are most effective in treating chronic diseases where the patient's general health and ability to resist an illness are important (Fulder 1988: 4). When people do consult alternative therapists for serious conditions, the vast majority of them also receive treatment for the same conditions from a doctor; however, most of those patients (72 per cent in Eisenberg *et al.* 1993) do not inform their doctor that they are also seeing alternative therapists (see also Sawyer *et al.* 1994). The medical profession has accused alternative medicine of encouraging petty complaints, self-absorption and unnecessary treatments (Easthope 1993), with a writer in the *Medical Journal of Australia*, the mouthpiece of the Australian Medical Association, stating that the alternative therapies 'medicalize discomforts which may be better regarded as essential parts of normal human experience' (Maddocks 1985: 549). Despite such a reluctance on the part of medical practitioners, however, there seems to be strong demand from patients for their doctors to provide them with alternative therapies (Himmel *et al.* 1993).

'She treats me like a person': therapeutic relationships in alternative therapies

The second dimension of the popular appeal of alternative medicine is the type of relationship it encourages between an active patient and a health-care practitioner who acts as a personal adviser rather than a superior. Alternative practitioners report that the patients they see are becoming more assertive consumers, in that they shop around more and consider themselves experts on their own bodies – they are on their own path to healing and want to be empowered to care for themselves by health-care 'consultants'. This has been borne out by studies of users of alternative medicine which have found them to be more active with regard to self-care than the general population and more assertive in relation to the professionals they consult (Sheehan 1984). The power dynamics in these alternative professional relationships are therefore very different to that traditionally encouraged by modern medicine. In one Sydney study, over 40 per cent of alternative medicine users cited the kind of interaction they had with alternative practitioners as an important difference from orthodox medicine, referring to 'a more caring attitude on the part of the alternative therapist', 'personalized and individualized attention' and 'better sharing of information' (Lloyd *et al.* 1993: 141–2). The medical profession have been taking note of this popular appeal and there have long been calls from within the establishment for medicine to take on board the use of such 'pleasant rituals and touching techniques' (as the medical profession patronizingly refers to this approach) in order to ease the discomfort and fears of their patients (Maddocks 1985: 549).

Studies of the health beliefs of users of alternative medicine suggest that they have more confidence in their own capacity for self-care and more faith in their ability to improve their health positively (Sheehan 1984: 75). One such study found that homeopathic patients considered lifestyle factors very important in determining health and engaged in proactive self-care practices more than did general practitioner patients. However, they appeared to take less notice of health messages from television and radio (Furnham and Bhagrath 1993: 239). This may stem from a preference for seeking out more detailed self-care advice from specialist practitioners, books and magazines while being more discriminating with regard to mainstream health information disseminated through mass media. Because alternative therapies see individual symptoms and many forms of illness as signs of underlying imbalance, as well as treating the specific issue, they are more likely to focus attention on the health of the person more generally, including their diet, emotional life, exercise, spiritual beliefs, and so on. In order to canvass this vast range of health-related information, consultations for alternative therapists are generally much longer than medical consultations.

Patients often report feeling that they are treated as a real person by alternative practitioners rather than a number or a walking medical condition. Of course, this attention to personal detail and counselling severely reduces the number of patients who can be seen, and the usual retort of medical practitioners is that they would love to be able to spend so much time providing an individualized service for each of their patients but they simply cannot afford to.

What they mean is that they do not want their income to drop to the income level of alternative therapists, which is on the whole considerably lower. Within alternative medicine there is the temptation for successful therapies with high patient demand to shorten their consultation times in order to see more patients, and such a tension can be seen between osteopathy and chiropractic. These are two very similar branches of manipulative therapy but the average consultation time of osteopathy in Australia is considerable longer than that of chiropractic. According to a 1985 Australian survey of chiropractors, their median gross income was A\$62 000, with roughly a third earning over A\$90 000, and a third earning under A\$49 000 (University of Queensland 1985: 20). According to these estimates of number of patients and fees charged, chiropractic incomes are similar to those of medical practitioners in private practice. Osteopaths, with their longer consultation times but similar fees, have lower incomes, and the resulting criticism of chiropractic practice is one of the main threads of the continuing tensions between osteopathy and chiropractic (O'Neill 1994).

Alternative therapies also express an interest in the spiritual dimension of illness and healing. They accuse medicine of actively undermining traditional forms of health care in which self-care practices were closely tied to spirituality, interpersonal relationships and more 'natural' ways of life. According to the literature surrounding contemporary alternative therapies, the healing process should facilitate and encourage a deeper level of introspection in the patient, who should use the therapeutic work as an opportunity to look inside their body for revelations concerning their own deep spiritual, psychological and emotional states. In practice, however, this emphasis on spirituality usually boils down to a heightened awareness of one's emotional and psychological state (Coward 1989: 74–5).

While advocates of alternative medicine stress that the way of life encouraged by dominant social forces is productive of modern ailments, the social determinants of health and illness are responded to in a very individualistic manner. To draw attention to the contribution of others or broader social contexts in the causation of illness is often seen as a form of 'negativity'. Alternative medicine has been criticized, most notably by Coward (1989), for fostering conservative ideologies of personal responsibility for health. Calls for action at the level of the broader context in which the individual's health is shaped are often deferred until after the condition is addressed at the individual level. The political changes which would be seen as 'progressive' by context-oriented public health approaches often meet with indifference from New Agers, for whom the notion of 'progress' is inseparable from the individual project of the cultivation of 'awareness' and the cumulative collective project of 'the evolution of consciousness'. They generally argue that while social economic and environmental factors are implicated in causing 'unwellness', individuals must pursue behaviour which minimizes the risks they face.

The nostalgia for living naturally

The third dimension of alternative medicine's current popularity is the perceived naturalness, and therefore safety, of its therapeutic interventions. A preference for natural remedies is widespread, and alternative therapies along with many other consumer goods and services have benefited from this (Lloyd *et al.* 1993; Siahpush 1999). Most alternative therapies place great emphasis on the body's capacity for self-healing and aim to enhance rather than bypass the natural healing forces of the body. Less technologically transformed medicinal substances are preferred, such as those derived from naturally occurring rather than synthetic compounds, and those closer to their natural state in preference to those humanly transformed (Coward 1989: 20). Because treatments usually aim only to stimulate the body's own self-healing capabilities, alternative therapies tend to use relatively weak and harmless remedies, compared with those employed by orthodox medicine. The medical monopoly on the use of surgery and most pharmaceuticals has also limited the alternatives to less invasive treatments. Despite this legal influence on their therapeutic practices, alternative medicines generally have a strong in-principle opposition to potentially harmful interventions in the body's natural processes.

In the eighteenth and nineteenth centuries, a common identity began to be forged between various unorthodox therapies, centred on a shared opposition to orthodox medicine. From the beginning of the nineteenth century, Samuel Hahnemann, the founder of homeopathy, referred to orthodox medicine as 'allopathy', a derogatory term which came to be used by many forms of alternative medicine to deride orthodox medicine. According to Hahnemann, allopathic medicine uses treatments which are supposed to counteract the symptoms produced by disease, while homeopathy uses substances which produce similar symptoms to the disease, in the belief that such substances encourage the body's own healing forces into action. Thus, for proponents of alternative medicine, the conflict between orthodox and unorthodox medicines came to be centred on whether the therapy worked with or against the body.

Modern medicine is still replete with militaristic imagery, its latest war being fought against cancer. The persistence of this traditionally masculine rhetoric has become more visibly a problem for medicine in light of the more peaceful and traditionally feminine values which have been associated with alternative medicine since the 1970s. A typical alternative medical critique of orthodox medicine describes it as

> a kind of divide and conquer mentality where you isolate the germs that are causing the symptoms and get rid of them. [...] Armies of doctors armed with an arsenal of pharmaceutical photon blasters and minutemen missiles, aided by battalions of specialists wielding high-tech scimitars [...] spare no expense in winning their battles and conquering new territories of exotic symptoms.
>
> (Tamura 1993: 17)

The professional self-care promotion which alternative therapists engage in has close ties with the natural health movement of the nineteenth century. While nineteenth-century natural health reformers such as Graham advocated healthy lifestyles, others heavily influenced by the same ideas developed therapeutic systems which broke drastically with traditional medical practice in order to align expert intervention with the body's own natural or God-given healing properties. The work of Andrew Taylor Still, founder of osteopathy, provides a good example of the way in which a 'nature religion' philosophy of self-healing was incorporated into professional practice and publishing. The founder of chiropractic, Daniel David Palmer, borrowed heavily from Still's work, but both of these 'inventors' merely systematized and institutionalized a body of lay bone-setting knowledge and practice which had been in existence in a less organized form for centuries (Hildreth 1942: 45; Gibbons 1979: 13; Gevitz 1982: 15–18). Still preferred to see himself as the discoverer of a science of divine origin, recounting in his 1898 autobiography how God's wisdom was passed to him:

> Twenty-four years ago, the 22nd day of June, at 10 o'clock, I saw a small light on the horizon of truth. It was put into my hand, as I understand, by the God of Nature. That light bore on its face the inscription: 'This is My medical library, My surgery and My obstetrics. This is My book with all the directions, instructions, doses, sizes, and quantities to be used in every case of sickness, and birth, the beginning of man; in childhood, youth and declining days.'
>
> (cited in Homola 1963: 121)

If God had created man in his own likeness, then the human body should be designed perfectly, and so any deviations from this perfection must be induced by man rather than God. Still believed that God would have designed man as a self-sufficient machine, containing all necessary therapeutic requirements. Drawing on his knowledge of mechanics, and believing that illness could not be due to bad design on the part of God, he proposed that illness was caused by the body's structure becoming maladjusted, as would happen to the machinery he had worked on. Illness could, according to his theory, be cured through structural adjustment by manipulating the bones.

Still inherited from his staunchly religious father a strong aversion to alcohol and, increasingly, all other drugs, which he came to hold in equal contempt. He believed that the body should be able to fix itself. In June 1874, he later reminisced, he had foreseen the end of technological medicine, and 'thought the sword and cannons of nature were pointing and trained upon our system of drug doctoring' (Still 1899: 13). Because, for Still, the composition and ordering of the body were intentional and reflected God's plan, the efforts of 'drug doctoring' to overpower the body or improve on natural processes was deeply suspect. Conversely, the therapeutic power of osteopathy lay in the ability to realize God's designs by manipulating the bones to restore the socially deformed or maladjusted body to the state which God intended. Still's radical attitude toward drugs in an era which favoured harsh drug treatments understandably caused some to label him a crank; however, he was able to draw upon a wide range of contemporary anti-pharmaceutical healing systems to create a systematic philosophy of osteopathy (Hildreth 1942: 14).

One of the most important of these was water cure, which involved using hot baths, hot packs, hot ears of corn and hot water bottles to produce an intense sweat which would carry toxins from the body (Hildreth 1942: 1). Drawing on such established and popular ideas, Still was able to explain in more detail the physical mechanisms which the manipulation of bones relied upon. The explanatory framework he established incorporated the popular belief that disease is caused by the build-up of toxins in the body. Although the form of the therapies differs widely, in this sense the understanding of the effects of these treatments was very similar. According to Still, the osteopath adjusts the body's framework

> so that all arteries may deliver blood to nourish and construct all parts. Also that the veins may carry away all impurities dependent upon them for renovation. Also that the nerves of all classes may be free and unobstructed while applying the powers of life and motion to all divisions, and the whole system of nature's laboratory.
>
> (Still 1899: 27–8)

Still saw disease as caused by the build-up and fermentation of impurities which nature intended should be routinely washed out of the body and discharged. The expulsion of impurities 'by way of the bowels, lungs, kidneys, and porous system' is controlled primarily, he states, by the nerves of the lymphatic system. By working particular nerves through spinal manipulation, the osteopath could help the body to eliminate toxins, preventing fermentation and eventual disease. The osteopath could tap into

> the power of nature to cure both old and young, by skillfully adjusting the engines of life so as to bring forth pure and healthy blood, the greatest known germicide [...] to conduct the vitalizing and protecting fluids to throat, lungs and all parts of the system, and ward off diseases as nature's God has indicated.
>
> (Still 1899: 15)

Still believed this vitalizing force is transmitted through the body via both the bloodstream and nerves and that the efficiency of transmission is determined by the degree of adjustment of the body's structural frame. The early research which he claimed led to his discoveries involved feeling for 'the speed, quality and heat' of the flow of blood beneath the skin. In 1870 he formulated his 'rule of the artery', which stated that 'whenever the circulation of the blood is normal, disease cannot develop because our blood is capable of manufacturing

all the necessary substances to maintain natural immunity against disease'
(Stanway 1980: 117).

Alternative therapies almost universally emphasize the body's self-regulating,
self-healing capacities, and believe that the role of the health-care practitioner is
to facilitate the body's self-healing process. Treatments aim at encouraging and
harnessing inherent healing energies, or host resistance, which operate to overcome illness. Symptoms are viewed in relation to the health status of the 'whole'
person, and are treated as indications of the nature of the imbalance in the
person's health. Symptoms provide an indication of the type of intervention
necessary to maximize the body's own attempts to return a state to equilibrium.
Consequently, pathologies are less likely to be explained in terms of a distinct
causal agent, as is the aspiration of orthodox medical explanation, but are
considered signs of systemic imbalance which can be treated effectively only by
working on the health of the person as a whole rather than treating the particular symptoms. This is of course not a new idea, as is attested by Voltaire's quip
that 'the art of medicine consists of amusing the patient while nature cures the
disease'. Many commentators on alternative medicine see this attempt to mobilize the self-healing capacities of the body as the primary common bond which
unites the diverse therapies, and the other commonalities which alternative therapies share are seen to derive from this central belief in self-healing (Fulder
1988: 3). In this sense, the view of the body within alternative medicine, as
derived from nineteenth-century Romanticism and natural health, has much
more in common with contemporary environmental consciousness than with
biomedical science.

Much of the popularity of alternative therapies comes from the way in which
they construct the body as requiring assistance in its self-healing processes only if
the 'natural' patterns of the body have been disrupted, or put out of balance.
Restoring this natural balance in the person's health requires the therapist and
the patient to take into account many facets of the person's lifestyle, depending,
of course, on the therapy in question. In locating the source of the imbalance or
disruption, 'modern' conceptual distinctions between spheres of the body or of
health give way to greater diagnostic and therapeutic connectivity between
spheres of behaviour, consciousness, health and environment.

Alternative therapies work with a broader definition of health than orthodox
medicine. Rather than an absence of symptoms, health is taken to mean a state
of complete physical and mental well-being in which the person's somatic, intellectual, emotional and spiritual faculties are working in a balanced and
harmonious manner so that a person is unlikely to become ill (Coward 1989: 74).
Attention to the whole person involves a more intense focus on emotions, diet,
exercise, sleeping habits, personal relationships. By contrast, the tendency of
mainstream health care to treat only the particular symptom or disease in isolation is seen as its central flaw. Because of this narrowness of focus, it is argued,
orthodox medicine both fails to deliver real health, and is responsible for much
unnecessary suffering, caused by side-effects and inhuman and uncaring treatment (Coward 1989: 7–8).

When considered in relation to Norbert Elias's work on the civilized body, this shift back to the 'natural body' seems paradoxical. For centuries in the West, social privilege has been associated with the cultivation of a controlled body, in which the 'base' aspects of embodiment have been banished by the upper classes. However, the Romantic nature which has been rediscovered is very different from the peasant nature against which the aristocracy defined itself. The alternative therapies' notion of nature is a long way also from a neo-Darwinian view of nature comprised of competing and hostile organisms, species or 'selfish genes', and by contrast almost entirely excludes violence and aggression (Coward 1989: 25). In alternative medicine's Romantic view of nature, the body is an 'innocent' entity worn down by a hostile artificial world. The presence of artificial substances in the body is seen as responsible for the production and accumulation of toxins in the body, and many methods of detox-ification are available for those who want to purge the artificial from their system. The purest and thus most natural of foods are fruit juices and purified water, and these are prescribed for those who are undergoing detoxification through fasting. Plants are generally considered less toxic than meat and animal products, whose status as both natural and potentially toxic causes much discus-sion on the virtues of vegetarianism.

While there are obvious continuities between earlier natural therapies and contemporary alternative therapies, I want to argue that there are also signifi-cant discontinuities between the historical predecessors of alternative medicine and the more recent manifestations since the 1970s. The recent therapies reflect a new set of attitudes to the nature of the person and the ideal therapeutic rela-tionship. The shared exclusion from state-sponsored health-care systems of alternative therapies since the nineteenth century has helped forge a long-standing sense of collective identity amongst the alternative medicines. This oppositional social milieu expanded and transformed rapidly with the height-ened health consciousness of the 1970s to comprise shared magazines, educational facilities and multi-therapeutic clinics. This close association with the counter-culture and a growing environmental consciousness increased the cohe-siveness of the range of excluded therapies and saw the application of a new 'holistic paradigm' as an over-arching philosophy of health and health care which reframed the older and more discrete philosophical systems of each distinct therapeutic system.

The post-1960s natural therapists found themselves culturally very different to the older natural therapists, who were often their teachers. The older generation of natural therapists were often people of iron will, used to being obeyed by their patients. They emphasized fasting, diet, elimination, clean living, godliness, high moral fibre and were often culturally conservative. The new generation were more 'counter-cultural' in their attitudes. They were more radical and anti-scien-tific in their outlook. Many of the new natural therapists had been influenced by the student movements of the late 1960s and the campaign against the Vietnam War, and saw alternative medicine as part of a new questioning attitude toward authority. For most alternative practitioners, a fundamental difference between alternative and orthodox medicine is the broader framing approach to the patient and to the causes and meanings of illness, which I will elaborate on below.

So far I have discussed only alternative medicine's interest in the body's capacity for self-healing as a non-conscious process which the body engages in 'naturally'. That is, if restored to its natural state, left alone and treated properly, the body knows what to do to regain health. But alternative medicine also uses the notion of self-healing to describe the self-active pursuit of positive health in which the patient is expected to be an active agent in all aspects of the healing process. The patient must seek a subjective understanding of the reasons for the illness and is encouraged to treat the introspection which treatment involves as a process of self-discovery (Fulder 1988: 5). Alternative therapists understand their role in the therapeutic process as helping patients to help themselves, in an instructional partnership characterized by mutual respect. The patient must be willing and motivated to change their behaviour to achieve a state of positive well-being before well-being can be achieved. As one advocate of 'the new health agenda' describes the message of alternative medicine, 'patients must become willing to invite wellness into their lives by ordering their daily living habits in conformity with the common sense rules of good health' (Carrol 1994: 49). As we shall see in the following section, a vast assortment of such 'common-sense rules' are substantiated with reference to romanticized views of a benevolent and virtuous nature.

How to live naturally

The most common means of rhetorically grounding highly detraditionalized contemporary self-care practices is to convince an audience of their 'natural-ness', expressing a nostalgia for more concretely organized ways of life. These claims act rhetorically to counter the disembedding tendencies of abstract self-care advice, based on technical expertise and communicated at a distance through disembodied communications, which often have the effect of further destabilizing one's ontological security.

Harvey and Marilyn Diamond's *Fit For Life* (1986), one of the top-selling self-care books since its publication, simplifies and popularizes the doctrine of 'Natural Hygiene', which the authors have reclaimed from nineteenth-century American natural health texts. Natural Hygiene's therapeutics are centred on eating practices, promising a complete system for 'the care and upkeep of the human body', purifying the body through diet. Natural Hygiene is both a way of living and an ideal form of embodiment, which emphasizes purity, beauty and serenity. The authors explain their first contact with the notion in these glowing terms:

> The first time I heard the term, I was staring into the face of the healthiest person *I* had ever met. One look at him and I knew he *had* to know some-thing about how to take care of his body. As I looked at his clear eyes,

radiant skin, serene demeanor, and well-proportioned body, I could not help but reflect on all the health professionals I had sought advice from in the past who did not exemplify the physical ideal any more than I did.

(Diamond and Diamond 1986: 13)

The man who knew how to take care of his body became a guru to Harvey Diamond on the basis of his appearance, which they saw as a sign of his expertise in self-management. And, just as the authors turned to a beautiful person, the public now turn to the beautiful people to learn how to manage their life. Beautiful celebrities market their own aerobics regimes, diets and semi-autobiographical self-help books. A brief glance at photographs of authors of the titles which fill the self-help section in any bookshop will reveal a group who are appear impossibly serene, contented and shiny. They smile and exude a studied air of warm goodwill. These are the faces of the saviours of postmodernity's lost souls – the faces who promise that health, happiness and full self-control are within your grasp and they are contained within the pages of this book.

Fit for Life, like many other contemporary natural health texts, draws on the teachings of the American natural health movement of the latter half of the nineteenth century. While medicine at that time was shifting away from the harsh treatments which characterized the first third of the century and was taking greater interest in diet and regimen, it was far surpassed in its embrace of natural methods by a vast array of anti-medical natural therapies which sought innovative techniques for using the healing power of nature. Unlike medical educators of the time and the medical self-help texts described above, these 'crusaders for fitness', as they have been called, posited an idealized state of health which was to be actively pursued.

The romanticization of nature is closely related to the increasing gravity of modernization risks, as Norbert Elias (1991a, 1991b) observed long before the current wave of environmental consciousness. As societies gain control of nature, including the biological processes of the body, the major threats and causes of insecurity are increasingly caused by the uncontrollable nature of other people's and states' actions. Nature, rendered relatively harmless in modernity, comes to be romanticized and treated nostalgically, and the natural body resurfaces in a positive form as the civilizing process becomes visible as a major constraint in itself. Nature comes to be seen in connection with the inner self, and 'artificial' social impediments are seen as restricting our 'authentic' inner 'nature' from being fully realized.

The natural health movement, which first gained popularity in something like its present form in the late nineteenth century, presents a strong counter-movement to the scientization of health and self-care. In the natural health movement, religious explanations gave way to natural explanations for health and illness. Writing soon after the turn of the twentieth century, William James referred to these nature religions as New Thought. The central tenet of this disparate array of therapeutic and religious practices, he observed, was that 'Nature, if only you will trust her sufficiently, is absolutely good' (W. James 1982:

80). In the nineteenth century, the appeal of nature was very much a reaction to the rapid technologization of life. As heavily refined white bread became popular in the United States, whole-grain alternatives were proclaimed by health reformers to have numerous health-promoting qualities. Not just whole-grain bread, but 'whole' foods of all sorts were promoted as natural and healthy.

A range of health movements popularized by personalities such as Sylvester Graham and John Harvey Kellogg, and therapeutic systems including herbalism, homeopathy, hydrotherapy and osteopathy, all shared a similar cultural milieu in the United States at that time. While there were substantial differences between them – in their mode of therapeutic practice, popularity and historical development – all of these combine elements of 'nature religion' with a preventive system of self-care practice and a related system of curative treatment. As with many more recent forms of alternative medicine, there is considerable overlap between proactive self-care and reactive self-treatment programmes – both involve undoing the damage caused by unhealthy lifestyles, restoring the person to a state of 'harmony with nature' so that the body's own healing powers can begin operating once more.

Many of these nineteenth-century movements were formed by deeply religious Christians who felt a need to expand their teachings into the realm of self-care practices, and so the relationship between God, nature, lifestyle and health pervades much of their self-care advice. The involvement of religious groups in health care and self-care issues takes a number of forms. Here I am elaborating on a framework developed by Catherine Albanese (1990: 121).

1   Religions may offer their own explanations for health and illness and feel threatened by or hostile towards scientific medicine's naturalistic explanations of these phenomena. In earlier periods Christian ethical systems had treated the freedom of their subjects as a freedom to diverge from the 'proper' path, and the church's teachings had revolved around keeping the flock on the straight and narrow. Being in the right, or following the way of God, was for the pre-modern Church a condition of the absence of independent decision-making consistent with following the customary patterns of life (Bauman 1993: 4). Sickness was often seen as a punishment for sin or lack of faith, or else as a test of one's faith.

2   A more minimalist role for religions is merely to console the ill and help them in the task of interpreting the meanings of illness. This is the attitude of the majority of modern religions, which accept a division of labour in the business of salvation between religious and health-care professionals.

3   Religions may see themselves as possessing their own healing powers which operate on a spiritual level out of reach of more materialist approaches to the body. They may see these techniques as either in conflict with or complementary to medical approaches. Prayer is an important part of the teaching of Christian responses to illness, while exorcism and charismatic healing persist uneasily at the fringes of most mainstream churches.

4   The fourth type of relationship between religion and health care is the development of self-care based on what Albanese (1990) has termed 'nature religion'. This was a form of religiosity in which caring for oneself and living 'naturally' constituted the central ritual enterprise for believers. Much contemporary self-care promotion has incorporated the nineteenth-century natural health movements' belief in the health-promoting properties of the 'natural'. The health reformers were innovative in treating the ordinary practices of followers as a matter of free choice among a range of options, and offered a choice between a Christian-natural lifestyle and one which was tainted by the ungodly artifice of mankind (modernity). Instead of seeing the normal pattern of life of the population as the true path contrasted with evil deviancies from the norm, these campaigners, in evangelistic fashion, saw the lifestyle of the majority of their audiences as in need of serious modification. The natural health movement, Albanese observes, consisted of 'injunctions and admonitions that, in effect, formed an ethical system for everyday life – to walk the path of "prevention" that, at least theoretically, led to fewer and fewer celebrations of the ritual cure' (Albanese 1990: 123).

Large sections of American Christianity changed their thinking about illness in the nineteenth century. Many came to see it as caused by the individual themselves rather than by God. God, they believed, had established natural laws for mankind, which it was the duty of the individual to conform to, and divergence from these laws resulted in illness. It followed that those who lived closest to nature would be nearest to perfect health. Joseph Wall, editor of the *Health Journal*, the prominent repository for Christian physiological thought, instructed:

> If man ever attains a heaven of happiness, he must do it by yielding obedience to the laws of his being, and coming into harmony with himself and the universe around him. If he does not do this, he will inevitably plunge himself into what may be justly called a hell of torment and misery.
>
> (cited in Albanese 1990: 126)

As more and more self-care techniques were developed, the natural health movement constructed an increasingly comprehensive ethical system for self-care and the conduct of everyday life. While the decision-making process was conceived as an individual one, the broader patterns of sickness were held to be caused by a widespread degeneration of social life which was straying from (God's) natural laws. The *Health Journal* repeatedly told its readers,

> The natural appetites of man – and through them all the higher faculties – having become perverted from their original simplicity, by an improper indulgence, and his liberty and happiness thus sacrificed by a departure from the plain and obvious laws of his nature, he can only regain his lost

paradise, by voluntarily yielding to the simple truth, and freely conforming
to the laws established in his constitution by his Creator.

(cited in Albanese 1990: 125–6)

The nineteenth-century advocates of nature religion warned that the ways of
God and nature had been undermined by modern 'indulgence' – a view which
was resurrected in the 1980s in the American religious Right's warnings of the
rise of 'permissive' lifestyles (B. Ehrenreich. 1989). The first issue of the
Vermont hydrotherapy magazine *Water Cure World* in 1860 illustrates this
Christian critique of 'social decay' vividly:

> We regard Man, in his primitive and natural condition as the most perfect
> work of God, and consider his present degenerated physical state as only the
> natural and inevitable result of thousands of years of debauchery and
> excess, of constant and willful perversions of his better nature, and the
> simple penalty of outraged physical law, which is as just and more severe
> than any other.

(cited in Albanese 1990: 137)

It was widely believed in the late nineteenth century that acquired characteristics were handed down to one's progeny. Improving one's health by living
according to God-given natural laws was seen not as a selfish course of action,
but as one which would benefit one's children and their children. Healthy
behaviour thus constituted an investment in long-term social change. The individual's responsibility was not only to themselves, but to the future of the race,
faced as it was with a choice between salvation and decay.

There is little difference between the explanatory frameworks of Christian
physiologists and secular natural therapists of the period. Consider, for example,
the theory of illness espoused by the *Homeopathic Advocate*, which centres on the
violation of natural laws. A sick person, it argued, is one who has 'through ignorance [...] violated some law of nature, and pain and sickness are the inevitable
result'. It is therefore

> of vast importance that we should all understand those laws which govern
> our own constitutions, and how to obey them in order to enjoy all the bless-
> ings designed by nature to flow from their obedience, as well as to escape the
> penalties attached to their infraction.

(cited in Albanese 1990: 134)

Although there is no reference to God as the author of natural laws, there are
nonetheless strong religious connotations in such a discussion of 'blessings' which
are 'designed' by nature.

One of the nineteenth-century natural health movement's most prominent
advocates, Sylvester Graham, had been a Presbyterian Minister for two years
before turning to lecturing for the Pennsylvania Temperance Society. While

following the established path of requiring total abstinence from alcohol in order to attain spiritual perfection, Graham also emphasized the deleterious physical effects of poor hygiene. He appropriated French physiologist François Broussais's recently published theory that repeated over-stimulation of tissue causes irritation and inflammation, especially in the stomach and intestines, and with this scientific foundation he proceeded to fill out a systematic account of the role of food and drink in causing illness and sustaining health (Whorton 1982: 41–3). 'Stimulation' had a dual meaning in American Protestant thinking at that time. In a physical sense, stimulation referred to the excitation and arousal of the flesh by touching, overt displays of sexuality, as well as by the consumption of rich foods and drink. In a moral sense, it was believed that excessive mental and emotional stimulation and excitement provided the psychic state in which a person's will was weakened to create susceptibility to sinful desires. According to historian James Whorton, by the 1830s 'the Victorian antipleasure principle was sufficiently far advanced as to have branded overstimulation, or nervous and mental excitation, as morally evil, the first step into a gradual descent into drunkenness and debauchery' (Whorton 1982: 43). Broussais's theory concerning the negative physiological effects of overstimulation fitted well into a Victorian culture in which animal desires and passions needed to be suppressed in order to promote godliness and good health.

A proper diet, according to Graham, would include foods with just enough stimulation to balance the vital force necessary for digestion. He argued that overly stimulating foods (those that had been modified from God's design by being purified or concentrated) would render them too nutritious and would result in irritation, inflammation and decreasing vitality (Whorton 1982: 48–9). Thus Graham ruled out meat, eggs, fresh milk, coffee, tea and pastries, instead advocating a diet filled with bland foods such as unrefined grains. He invented the high-fibre 'Graham cracker' to fill the gap in the market he had just created (Gevitz 1982: 11). However, Graham's was not a purely dietary approach to positive health. Like many other Protestant health reformers, he targeted restrictive or improper dress, sexual permissiveness and prescription medicines as causes of illness. Graham's lectures and books argued for these modern evils to be replaced with regular exercise, bathing and fresh air (Gevitz 1982: 10).

The appeal of the natural in this period needs to be understood in the context of the detraditionalization of self-care practices then taking place in the United States. The food industry was increasingly refining and processing existing foods and producing many novel foods, so the range of dietary choices was beginning to expand rapidly. These natural-religious self-care philosophies provided an ethical basis for dietary choice to those anxious about cultural change. But they did not merely reaffirm traditional practices. These more abstract dietary regimes themselves added to the range of options available. From the late nineteenth century and early twentieth century this nature-religious advice about the virtues of traditional foods and purifying practices such as hydrotherapy began to be swamped by the increasing amounts of commercial advertising of modern foods, and the appeal to the natural became just one of many themes in the proliferation of commercial dietary advice.

By the early twentieth century, the most prominent health reformers had a greater interest in more vigorous pursuits and in strengthening the body than in 'hygienic' campaigns. A good illustration of this trend is provided by the magazine started in the United States by Bernarr Macfadden in 1899 called *Physical Culture*, whose motto was 'Weakness is a Crime'. This was a new kind of publication full of articles and illustrations, which, like his many books, educated the reader in the performance of physical exercises, in order to attain and enjoy what he called 'health plus' (Whorton 1988: 76). Macfadden poetically explained what he meant by health at the beginning of his five-volume *Encyclopedia of Physical Culture* (1914):

> Health means vim, vigor, snap and energy. Health means clarity and strength of mind; purity and beauty of soul. The healthy person is unconscious of discomfort; he rises superior to it – is absolutely the monarch of all he surveys. He dominates life instead of allowing it to dominate him. [...] He is a unit – a being – a man, whole, complete, vigorous, perfect, happy – because healthy. To such a man work is a joy; obstacles but opportunities for endeavor, difficulties but a means for enlarged triumph. [...] Health is what gives manhood to man; womanhood to woman.
>
> (cited in Whorton 1988: 77)

There are several interesting features here which reveal a transition taking place from the dominant form of nineteenth-century self-care promotion. Firstly, health is conceived as an ideal state attained through physical work upon one's self. It is seen as the ideal end-point of self-improvement rather than a prior natural state which can be regained through cleansing or purification. Secondly, in stark contrast to the stern anti-indulgence ethic of nineteenth-century Protestantism, in the physical fitness movements of the early twentieth century, health is celebrated as a means of attaining physical pleasure, happiness and power over one's body and life. Macfadden celebrated bodily pleasure, beauty and virility, publishing books with titles such as *Muscular Power and Beauty*, *Hair Culture*, *Superb Virility of Manhood* and *Marriage: A Lifelong Honeymoon*. Sexual vigour, he believed, was the foundation of manhood and womanhood and the necessary starting point for all other health gains. His licentiousness and active opposition to what he called 'the curse of prudishness' got him arrested in 1907 over an issue of *Physical Culture* which included an allegedly 'obscene' article on the modes of transmission of venereal disease (Whorton 1988).

James Whorton sees already in early twentieth-century popular health movements the roots of a late twentieth-century narcissistic and self-absorbed self-care. He laments the passing of the earlier (Protestant) ethic which saw health as a means to personal efficiency and commercial accomplishment, which he believes had given way to a narrower concern with individual well-being through physical and emotional self-actualization (Whorton 1988: 80). Where

the religious advocates of natural health argued in moral terms for the importance of returning to purity, the secular health advocates were more inclined to
emphasize health as a pleasurable state. Strength, vitality, fitness and the bodily
pleasure which may have resulted from them were seen by the earlier
campaigners as signs of the correctness of the lifestyle, as rewards which ensued
from following the true path. To the early twentieth-century campaigners for
health, fitness and its performative and sensory benefits were ends in themselves.

Already, in the early twentieth century, we can see a yearning for a return to
more natural, less abstracted, ways of caring for the self that were at that time
perhaps subcultural but which had become thoroughly mainstream by the end of
the century. Like 'health', the term 'nature' now carries a package of interwoven
meanings, and natural techniques for the care of the self promise to help the
user return to a more raw, pristine and untainted form of embodiment, at the
same time as natural self-care promises low-risk courses of action (because
nature appears harmless to people who live in cities). Following a natural path,
apparently, is also the best way to 'release' one's inner reserve of vigour,
promising to enhance one's capacity for self-motivation, which is a primary
requirement for the successful self-management of autonomous individuals.

5 Self-care and anti-institutional politics

Before sickness came to be perceived as an organic or behavioural abnormality, he [*sic*] who got sick could still find in the eyes of the doctor a reflection of his own anguish and some recognition of the uniqueness of his suffering. Now, what he meets is the gaze of a biological accountant engaged in input/output calculations. His sickness is taken from him and turned into an institutional enterprise. His condition is interpreted according to a set of abstract rules in a language he cannot understand. He is taught about alien entities that the doctor combats, but only just as much as the doctor considers necessary to gain the patient's co-operation. Language is taken over by the doctors: the sick person is deprived of meaningful words for his [*sic*] anguish, which is thus further increased by linguistic mystification.

Ivan Illich, *Medical Nemesis* (1976: 175)

In the 1970s, many like Illich proclaimed self-care as the means for overcoming the disempowering dependency on professional-institutional health care. In their enthusiasm for active self-care, these critics of medicalization expressed a nostalgia for more concrete forms of self-care and overlooked the ways in which lay knowledge was being rapidly reconstituted through self-activating forms of professional practice and disembodied forms of integration. Sociology, since it first turned its attention to health in the 1950s, treated institutionalized health care as primarily an agent of social control. Self-care, then, was seen by many as a way of re-empowering individuals in the face of the alienating and deadening effects of rationalized medicine which Illich describes above. It is worth tracing back the construction of the position of the patient in relation to professional-institutional care in order to show the intellectual context in which the anti-institutional politics of self-care developed.

Parsons' passive patients

Medical sociology started to become established within American sociology departments in the 1950s and 1960s, at which time Samuel Bloom's *The Doctor and His Patient* was often a central text and Talcott Parsons' concept of the 'sick role' was central to the discipline. Early sociological interest in health, such as

Parsons', was not generally concerned with the subjective experience of health, and, when theorizing illness behaviour, tended to treat the medical practitioner as the only active agent in health care. Parsons' concept of the sick role described the manner in which patients were required to surrender aspects of their autonomy in return for treatment and exemption from social expectations. Since this time there has been a steady development of interest in the subjective domain of health and illness in the social and behavioural sciences.

Although Parsons' description of the sick role has been much criticized, his broader theoretical approach to health and illness conceived in terms of deviance and social control has endured in both mainstream and critical strands of the sociology of health (McEwen *et al.* 1983). Parsons used the terms 'health' and 'illness' in a functional sense, to designate a capacity or incapacity to partici-pate actively in the social system. Health, from this perspective, is 'the state of optimum capacity of an individual for the effective performance of the roles and tasks for which he [*sic*] has been socialized'. Likewise, sickness is defined as a 'generalized disturbance of the capacity of the individual in normally expected role or task performance' (Parsons 1958: 176). Parsons' functionalist approach was not interested in the subjective experience of health and illness. Failure to accept medical authority, he argued, would cause one to be seen as either a hypochondriac or in denial. He saw illness as a state of deviance, or disfunction-ality, and so understood the medical and social assistance given to the ill as a pressure to return to a state of functionality. Parsonian functionalism's overem-phasis on systemic imperatives thus began a tradition in the sociology of health in which health care (and especially medicine) was seen as primarily an institu-tion of social control.

Parsons argued that being sick constitutes a distinct social role because an individual in the condition is subject to a number of institutionalized behavioural expectations in modern Western societies. Unlike other social roles, which are dependent on one's social position in some way, any individual may fall into the sick role regardless of their social status in other respects. The key aspects of the sick role are as follows:

1 The sick person is exempted from a range of normal obligations. The exemption from normal role responsibilities is both a right and an obliga-tion, which is sometimes forced upon those not considered well enough to carry out their functions. The level of legitimate exception is dependent on the seriousness of the illness.

2 The sick person is not held responsible for their condition. While on occa-sion the patient may bear responsibility for the onset of an illness, they are even then not generally held responsible for its continuation (Parsons 1951: 436–7; Twaddle 1979: 44–5). Once a person is sick, regardless of the reasons for their illness, they are deemed to be in need of help and unable to be held responsible for their own care, as their condition is not able to be changed by an act of will.

3 Illness, or functional incapacity, is socially defined as undesirable, and an obligation is placed on the sufferer to want to get well. The privileges sanctioned in (1) and (2) are subject to this motivation to recovery, and conditional upon the appropriate reactive self-care of the sufferer.

4 The patient is obliged to seek help from and cooperate with professionals. The obligatory motivation to get well must be followed up by help-seeking behaviour. The intervention of professionals serves to legitimate one's claim to exemption from normal responsibilities.

The sick role entails both an abrogation of responsibilities and exemption from social obligations, but this is conditional upon a motivation on the part of the patient to participate in a therapeutic regime. The sick role theory sees positive motivations to get well as unconsciously carried systemic imperatives. Sickness, according to Parsons (1958), is by definition a condition for which the person cannot be held responsible. He argues that positive motivations to health are a result of the functional imperatives of the social system. The strong health-seeking behaviour of Americans, he believes, is related to the 'activism' of the American value system. In a society in which personal achievement, and the behavioural and attitudinal characteristics which are thought to underlie achievement, are thoroughly entrenched, there is a strong connection between the motivation to effective achievement and the motivation to health which is a precondition of such striving (Parsons 1958: 183).

As well as legitimating claims for special consideration, medicine imposes other forms of disincentive on the sick. They are forced into a condition of dependence on others, isolated from other sufferers lest they develop a camaraderie, a collective positive identification with the sick role (as does the delinquent gang in relation to criminal deviance).

> The conditional legitimation of the sick person's status [...] places him [*sic*] in a special relation to people who are not sick, to the members of his family and to the various people in the health services, particularly physicians. This control is part of the price he pays for his partial legitimation, and it is clear that the basic structure resulting is that of the dependence of each sick person on a group of non-sick persons rather than of sick persons on each other. This is in itself highly important from the point of view of the social system since it prevents the relevant motivations from spreading through either group formation or positive legitimation. [...] the sick role not only isolates and insulates, it also exposes the deviant to reintegrative forces.
>
> (Parsons 1951: 312–13)

This functional explanation of the experience of illness is rather thin. The sick were indeed isolated from one another in Parsons' time, and to a lesser extent are still, but this was primarily due to the tendency for people in modern societies to get sick individually, rather than with a number of people they know already. Once sick, there is little opportunity to meet others in the same condition, given that most sick people stay at home and those who are admitted to hospital are usually not in the mood for socializing. Parsons is only able to mount an argument concerning systemic imperatives in order to explain this phenomenon.

The role of therapeutic agencies, according to Parsons, is the recovery of the 'capacity for full and satisfactory functioning in a system of social relationships' (Parsons 1975: 258). The health-care system is seen as a mechanism of social control which works to increase motivation to recovery and reduce resistance to therapeutic efforts. This view of medicine was later taken up by critics of medicine, who saw it as an insidiously manipulative apparatus. Andrew Twaddle observed that in contrast to other forms of deviance, 'the sick person is defined as desiring conformity and, as a result, the sick person is seen as more likely to seek out the agents of social control and to actively work with them toward the goal of behavioural conformity' (Twaddle 1979: 198). In the 1970s Marxist critics of medicalization drew heavily on Parsons to criticize the individualizing effects of the medical construction of the patient, arguing that the adoption of the sick role 'relieves strains which otherwise could become a focus of dissatisfaction and conflict, it becomes a conservative (and sometimes counter-revolutionary) mechanism inhibiting social change' (Waitzkin and Waterman 1974: 35). They echoed Parsons in suggesting that medicine conceives of health primarily as a measure of the productive capacity of patients, and that the medical profession was simply carrying out the systemic requirement to maintain the well-being of individuals that is necessary in order to ensure that workers remain productive and make minimal demands on the welfare system. As we shall see below, many critics of medicalization accepted Parsons' functionalist analysis of medicine, but are critical of the social control which they believe medicine exercises.

Parsons' account of the dissemination of self-care advice by doctors ignores pre-existing 'lay' health beliefs and practices. Instead, he emphasizes the powerlessness of the patient in the face of professional-institutional authority. Parsons describes the way in which the doctor and patient are bound in a common task – the doctor is obliged to put the patient's welfare above all other interests, and the patient is obliged to comply and cooperate with the doctor (Parsons 1951: 438–9). The patient is in a vulnerable position, and Parsons notes a very strong feeling against exploitation of the sick (Parsons 1951: 43-5). The powerlessness of the patient and lay associates is not able to be willed away by democratically minded reformers (as he reiterated decades later) and is inevitable for a number of reasons. The patient's vulnerability is intrinsic to the relationship and has several dimensions. According to Parsons, patients and their lay associates are:

(a) in need of help, not responsible for own condition, cannot will themselves better, entitled to help;
(b) largely ignorant with regard to what needs to be done, and so reliant on the technically trained;

(c)   emotionally upset because of their suffering and frustrated due to incapaci-
tation. Because it is difficult for the patient to act rationally in this state, they
are vulnerable to persisting irrational beliefs and practices (Parsons 1951:
440–6, 1975).

Rational medicine, in Parsons' view, is opposed only to the prior irrationality
of its patients, which they are prone to revert to when under stress. In this
approach, Parsons is simply restating the view medicine had of itself as an agent
of demystification. This was perhaps the peak of popular respect for medicine,
and for science in general, in the West. Medical science promised to eradicate
the 'superstitious' explanations and treatments of traditional societies, which it
derogatorily (but perhaps rather accurately) referred to as old wives' tales. As the
bearer of professional-institutional power over the body, it made strategic sense
for it to deny the prior existence of effective lay health beliefs and practices.
Theorists of medicine like Parsons, however, should be able to see through this
medical rhetoric.

In merely restating the prevailing view of medicine as rolling back the ignorance and irrationality of the population, Parsons does not capture the
complexity of the patient's interaction with the professional. Thomas Szasz (later
to become a prominent anti-psychiatrist) and Marc Hollander sought to improve
on Parsons by distinguishing three types of doctor–patient relationships:
activity–passivity, guidance–cooperation and mutual participation. They argued
that each of these is appropriate to particular situations, dependent upon the
nature of the disease being treated and the type of patient (Szasz and Hollander
1956). Activity–passivity describes a situation in which the patient is unable to
participate in treatment due to the traumatic nature of the illness and the condition of emergency, requiring the practitioner to take almost complete
responsibility for the patient. Guidance–cooperation describes what the authors
see as the normal state of affairs in medical practice. The patient, by seeking
help and accepting the superiority of the doctor's knowledge, allows the doctor
to be in a position of authority. Both remain active participants in the relationship but the patient is expected to respect and obey the doctor's instructions.
Mutual participation is the usual state of affairs in treating chronic illness, where
the patient must manage their own conditions. The medical practitioner plays
the role of consultant in relation to the self-care of the patient, who is experienced and knowledgeable in relation to the illness. This form of relationship is
based on equality and is essentially foreign to medicine, the authors argue;
however, they note that 'the greater the intellectual, educational, and general
experiential similarity between physician and patient, the more appropriate and
necessary this model of therapy becomes' (Szasz and Hollander 1956: 587).
Szasz and Hollander's framework provides a useful starting point in understanding the level of active participation a patient is able to have in relation to
professional-institutional care. In some circumstances patients are necessarily
more dependent than in others. Emergency care necessitates a very different
relationship than does dealing with less incapacitating conditions and chronic

illnesses. Szasz and Hollander encourage doctors to promote active self-care by delegating some diagnostic and therapeutic responsibilities to patients (see also Williamson and Danaher 1978: 100). Medicine did not embrace this advice for it had too much faith in its own expertise to treat seriously the ill-informed views of its patients. It was only later, when patients had access to a plethora of health advice from the print and electronic media, that doctors were forced to acknowledge their more abstractly informed patients as active participants in their own care.

Early interest in lay health care

Things began to change when medical sociologists attempted to demonstrate the role played by patients themselves in interpreting and acting upon their illnesses. They were interested in the cultural determinants of reactive self-care, and especially the relationship between self-treatment decisions and professional health care. With the increasing influence of psychology and sociology in public health research in the post-war period, health behaviour came to be understood as the result of a person's beliefs rather than being natural or instinctual (Armstrong 1988: 16). In 1954, for example, a researcher advocating the study of parents' responses to their children's poliomyelitis vaccination stated that, '[u]sing the technics of social science research, it would seem fruitful to investigate further the methods of reaching and influencing those segments of the population which tend to be non-participants in such public health programs' (cited in Armstrong 1988: 16). These researchers were primarily concerned with understanding the factors which influenced public compliance with medical interventions.

Sociological interest in popular health beliefs can be traced back to Earl Koos' 1954 book, *The Health of Regionsville: What the People Thought and Did About It.* In this study, Koos' team interviewed 500 families over a four-year period in an unspecified American town. Since that time, surveys of health attitudes and experiences have been carried out widely by medicine and social science (Armstrong 1984: 740). Sociological studies in the 1960s drew both on survey-based health attitude research amassed by epidemiologists and on anthropological research on traditional belief systems. At the most general level, these surveys assess pervasive attitudes about what factors people believe are responsible for maintaining well-being or causing illness. On a more phenomenological level, the researchers undertaking these studies were interested in the way in which people interpret their own bodily states and to what extent they act upon troubling conditions by seeking help from others, whether family, friends or professional services – how they make decisions about whom to consult, when to seek help, what type of care is required, and so on. The pervasiveness of the experience of symptoms soon led to a consensus that the health-care system only comes in contact with the 'tip of the iceberg' of illness and that more than 75 per cent of illness episodes are not dealt with by professionals (Last 1963: 13). There was, however, little interest in proactive self-care or lifestyles at this time.

In light of this research, the dominant sick role theory was repeatedly criticized for overstating the power of the medical profession in shaping the experiences of the sick. Eliot Freidson argued that social acceptance of and support for the sick person, which Parsons had considered dependent on the patient's cooperation with medical authority, was actually more dependent on the sick person showing symptoms and behaviour which made sense to those around them in terms of their own lay concepts of illness (Freidson 1970: 289; Turner 1987: 45). Freidson (1961) coined the term 'lay referral systems' to described the processes by which people seek to understand their bodily states themselves and then in consultation with others before any professional advice is sought. Within the lay referral system Freidson distinguished broader lay cultural influences from lay networks of advice, which are networks of personal influence. He charted the ways in which people first consulted friends, family, neighbours, acquaintances with some health knowledge, for advice on troubling health issues, and, when needing to consult professionals, based their consultation decisions on advice or instructions from others. The lay cultural influences 'discovered' by Freidson are shared by communities through face-to-face integration and had been only partially reconstituted by professional-institutional knowledge. Interaction with other lay people usually precedes interaction with professionals and powerfully frames the person's experience both of professional care and of their illness.

Irving Zola (1966) argued that subjective interpretations of the meaning and seriousness of symptoms differed markedly between social groups. Zola's work showed that not only were cultural factors important in the aetiology of various diseases, predisposing certain groups to risks and influencing the progression of the disease, but cultural factors and ethnicity in particular were important in the subjective interpretation of bodily states, the presentation of symptoms to professionals and their descriptions of them. These researchers were interested in which symptoms were considered serious, causing people to seek treatment, and which were tolerated as trivial or normal. These decisions were found to be culturally determined, so sickness came to be seen as a social constructed category rather than an objective fact. Other studies focused on the cultural construction of 'normal' body states and found that many 'symptoms' were largely ignored in some social groups as normal (Williamson and Danaher 1978: 45–7).

The lay beliefs revealed by these early ethnographic studies and surveys were predominantly 'folk' conceptions, in that they were contained within oral cultures and were communicated through face-to-face interaction and in a setting of face-to-face integration. These were contrasted with the professional knowledge systems of medicine, in which the practitioner acts as a representative of an abstract and impersonal body of knowledge which seeks to replace existing lay beliefs with more scientific understandings and create a distrust of folk knowledge in order to increase reliance on professional services. This was a conflict which was played out both on a societal level and in every medical encounter, between traditional (lay) and modern (professional and scientific) knowledge systems. Elliot Mishler (1981), for example, describes this divide as two separate discourses – the voice of medicine and the voice of the lifeworld – and argues that interactions between practitioners and patients should strive to achieve a balance between the two. This type of approach acknowledges that the patient, too, draws on a body of knowledge through which they interpret their own body and from within which they interact with professional expertise.

This lay–expert distinction has been criticized for not acknowledging that experts also draw on social knowledge and that the patient may draw on expertise of their own. Postmodernist writers tend to describe a plurality of discourses interrupting one another, and all speaking in both medical and social voices through both patients and practitioners (Silverman 1987; Fisher 1991). This pluralism denies that there are contradictory interests involved in the therapeutic relationship, instead arguing that the interests of both are served by effective communication. This view has been widely incorporated into the education of health-care practitioners, who are encouraged to realize that they also bring with them culturally determined views, and that they should be open to questioning and listening, and should encourage patients to participate in a dialogue with them about their health. We should take on board this observation that the lay–expert divide is not clear-cut, but there is no escaping the fact that professionals' power derives from a more abstract form of expertise which is fundamentally different to lay knowledge systems communicated at the face-to-face level. Both expert (institutionalized) and lay (face-to-face) knowledges become increasingly abstracted with a society now framed by disembodied modes of practice.

New Left critiques of medicine

Throughout the 1960s and 1970s the Left was more concerned with reforming institutional health care than promoting self-care. There was a strong individualistic anti-institutional politics within the New Left, especially in the US, which was expressed famously in the Students for a Democratic Society's 1962 Port Huron Statement. The statement defines human beings as 'infinitely precious and possessed of unfulfilled capacities for reason, freedom and love. Men have unrealized potential for self-cultivation, self-direction, self-understanding and creativity' (Goodheart and Curry 1992: 198). These beliefs fed into the Left counter-culture's fascination with reflexive self-care techniques of many kinds, from meditation and drug use to vegetarianism and yoga. While these alternative self-care techniques were becoming increasingly popular, radical and Marxist critiques of mainstream medicine in the late 1960s and early 1970s focused predominantly on the systematic exploitation of consumers by providers of health care and unequal access to services. Their aim was generally not to change the type of health care being offered but to extend the availability and equitable distribution of conventional medical services. There were very public protests at American Medical Association Conventions in this period, with the medical profession being accused of genocide by treating favoured wealthy clientele better and by focusing resources on the diseases of the rich (cancer, heart disease, stroke) while ignoring the diseases of the poor (malnutrition, high infant mortality) (Zola 1972). These challenges were not generally against the medical model of care but against the economic determinism of the health-care system, which distorted the objectivity of medical need.

Some Marxist critiques focused on the individualism of medical practice in light of the social causation of illness. Waitzkin and Waterman saw medicine as acting on behalf of an expansionary state which acts to alleviate the contradictions of capitalism in order to make the system run more smoothly. Medicine acts to draw attention away from the social and political bases of health by focusing on individual bodies through the biomedical paradigm. 'Insofar as adoption of the sick role relieves strains which otherwise could become a focus of dissatisfaction and conflict', they argue, 'it becomes a conservative (and sometimes counter-revolutionary) mechanism inhibiting social change' (Waitzkin and Waterman 1974: 35). At the same time it propounds ideologies of individual responsibility for health and puts a high moral value on the social usefulness and productiveness of health, so that well-being of the individual is necessary in order to ensure that workers remain productive while at the same time healthy workers place less burden on the welfare arm of the system. On the whole, liberal and radical critics agreed on the unjust distribution of health care but diverged in assigning causes. Liberals tended to blame poor organization, and the lack of affordable health insurance for the poor, while the Left blamed the system of private ownership, arguing for the establishment or improvement of public health systems. However, they both supported the expansion of medicine as an improvement on prior forms of health care.

The critique of medicalization

A number of writers in the 1970s responded to the popularity of non-medical forms of health care and anti-institutional critiques of medicine (including the anti-psychiatry movement of the late 1960s) by criticizing the deeper social, cultural and subjective effects of the expansion of medical power in the twentieth century (R. Fox 1988). The most influential of these was Ivan Illich, whose book *Medical Nemesis* contrasts self-care with 'heteronomous' institutional care. To medicine he applied his general argument that the institutionalization and professionalization of spheres of life undermine autonomous action by lay people which the institutions were originally intended to supplement and on which their success relies (Illich 1976). 'Nemesis' is an ancient Greek term referring to the vengeance wrought by the Gods upon hubris, or the aspirations of mortals to the attributes of gods through heroism. In avoiding technocratic terms for this phenomenon, Illich sought to distance himself from those who posit bureaucratic and technocratic solutions for the problems in health care. He believed that 'the *reversal of nemesis* can come only from within man and not from yet another managed (heteronomous) source depending once again on presumptuous expertise and subsequent mystification' (Illich 1976: 44). As we shall see, Illich, like many others, failed to comprehend the importance of disembodied 'heteronomous' sources in shaping the exercise of 'autonomous' self-care in the latter part of the twentieth century.

Illich argued that nature is fundamentally resistant to medical attempts to control the body technologically. In short, human frailty, he reminded us, is inescapable. Medical technological remedies which attempt to transcend the frailty of the body inevitably cause iatrogenic problems, that is, side-effects which are caused by medical treatment itself. Medical nemesis is the cumulative outcome of these side-effects which result from the desire of medicine to provide technological solutions to issues which are social in nature (such as stress) or are unavoidable aspects of the human condition (such as pain). Illich argued that medical nemesis can only be remedied through the 'recovery' of mutual self-care coupled with limits upon the legal, political and cultural power of medicine.

He argued that the counter-productivity of institutionalized health care is not an isolated phenomenon but a manifestation of a more generalized crisis across all sectors of industrialized societies (Illich 1976: 215). This is the tendency of institutions to undermine the qualities that they were intended to promote, that is, 'industrially generated destruction of those environmental, social, and psychological conditions needed for the development of non-industrial or non-professional use values. Counterproductivity is the result of an industrially induced paralysis of practical self-governing activity' (Illich 1976: 217). Professional-institutional health care transforms people into passive consumers of their own health rather than producers of it. Cultural resources which maintain health and which allow people to deal with suffering are eroded. As the ability to live and cope with impairment and pain is lost, people come to rely on professionals for a wider variety of crises and the growth in medical services cannot keep up with the growth in demand.

Illich labels counterproductivity in the health sphere as iatrogenesis, a term commonly used to refer to illnesses caused by doctors. Social iatrogenesis is the impairment of health due to the 'socio-economic transformations which have been made attractive, possible, or necessary by the institutional shape health care has taken' (49). The professionalization of health care has created a 'radical monopoly' in which medicine not only corners the market but also restricts and disables people from healing themselves, for example by placing legal restrictions on access to self-medication. This expropriation of health out of the hands of each person and into the hands of a trained profession also has the effect of de-legitimizing claims by ordinary people against the sickening effects of their environment, food, work, and so on. Medicine thus both worsens and at the same time obscures the social conditions which make people sick.

> An advanced industrial society is sick-making because it disables people from coping with their environment and, when they break down, it substitutes a 'clinical' prosthesis for the broken *relationships*. People would rebel

against such an environment if medicine did not explain their biological disorientation as a defect in their health, rather than as a defect in the way of life which is imposed on them or which they impose on themselves. The assurance of personal political innocence that a diagnosis offers the patient serves as a hygienic mask that justifies further subjection to production and consumption.

(Illich 1976: 174)

Illich and other critics of medical expansionism were following in the footsteps of the anti-psychiatrists. They wanted to show that this process was not unique to mental health and so sought to broaden the critiques of psychiatric diagnosis beyond psychiatry (Szasz 1961; Foucault 1965; Leifer 1969). 'Therapeutic interventions have two faces', wrote prominent anti-psychiatrist Thomas Szasz in his influential book *The Myth of Mental Illness*: 'one is to heal the sick, the other is to control the wicked. [...] Psychiatric diagnoses are stigmatizing labels, phrased to resemble medical diagnoses and applied to persons whose behavior annoys or offends others' (cited in J. Ehrenreich 1978: 5–6). Illich and Zola pointed out that with the medicalization of everyday life, in which the labels 'healthy' and 'ill' become relevant to ever-widening aspects of human existence, medicine is becoming a major mechanism for social control (Zola 1972: 487). They criticized the tendency for professional intervention to be extended via 'diagnostic imperialism' to all spheres of life, so that madness, depression, old age and reproduction become primarily medical problems. Eliot Freidson (1970) had earlier described how the medical profession has first claim to jurisdiction over the label of illness and anything to which it may be attached, irrespective of its capacity to deal with it effectively. Since the early twentieth century, more and more embodied states once considered normal aspects of life (such as ageing and reproduction) or considered as character flaws (alcohol and drug addictions) have become medical conditions. Because of the success of this expansionism, doctors are increasingly sought out for help by those with interpersonal and social problems (Zola 1972: 496). As the cultural meaning of 'health' expands, reflecting medical diagnostic imperialism, medicine is in a position, Zola argues, 'to exercise great control and influence about what we should and should not do to attain that "paramount value"' (Zola 1972: 498). These writers also shared with anti-psychiatrists such as Szasz and R.D. Laing a desire to redress the power imbalance between health-care professionals and patients (Laing 1965; Moorhouse 1969).

Zola's political concern is that the popular desire for health tends to heighten the power of medicine to enforce a particular notion of health and to reconstitute life in line with quite narrow and expertly (rather than democratically) determined therapeutic requirements. Support for medicalization has been in part based on the perceived demystification of illness, and the corresponding shift from religious interpretations to expert knowledge which diminished moral scrutiny and individual blame for one's health. Against those who argue that the medical model has lifted the moral condemnation of the individual, Zola points out that from the doctor's perspective this abrogation of personal blame is dependent upon the patient's full acceptance of and cooperation with the authority of the doctor over that patient's condition. This conditional sympathy is of course a central feature of Parsons' description of the sick role. Where Zola departed from Parsons was in pointing out that issues of personal responsibility which were once diminished by developments within biomedical thought (such as the germ theory of illness, heredity, etc.) were re-emerging, with new interest in the relationship between psychological states and physical states (notable with the interest in stress at the time he was writing). Zola was witnessing the beginnings of trends within medical knowledge itself which 'bring man [*sic*], *not* bacteria to the center of the stage and lead thereby to a re-examination of the individual's role in his own demise, disability and even recovery' (Zola 1972: 491). The relationship between lifestyle and disease supports medical intervention in previously irrelevant aspects of the sick person's life. The 'extension into life' is especially pronounced in treating chronic conditions and in preventive medicine which requires the doctor to attempt to change 'the habits of a patient's lifetime – be it of working, sleeping, playing or eating' (Zola 1972: 493).

A number of conservative writers in this period were critical of medicalization for much the same reasons. In 1975, Leon Kass argued in the conservative American journal *The Public Interest* that by aspiring to assist in the pursuit of happiness, medicine is pursuing misguided and unattainable aims. Psychiatric interventions to improve patients' emotional state, *in vitro* fertilization, abortion on demand and cosmetic surgery put the medical profession in a position in which they are called on to make moral and social decisions for which their technical training does not equip them. Kass specifically criticized the World Health Organization's broad definition of health ('a state of complete physical, mental and social well-being, and not merely the absence of disease or infirmity', WHO 1946) for being beyond the reasonable scope of medical practice. A second false aim of medicine, according to Kass, is that of behavioural modification in order to create more obedient or virtuous subjects. Doctors, he argued, lack the authority and competence to deal with issues such as criminality and anti-social behaviour. In this, Kass is in agreement with Left anti-psychiatrists, but his prescription of how these social issues should be dealt with is very different, stating that these are jobs for 'parents, policemen, legislators, clergymen, teachers, judges' as well as the individuals themselves and the community as a whole (Kass 1975: 14–15). He stresses personal responsibility for one's own health as an alternative to further medicalization, arguing for very limited state responsibility in the provision of medical services and public health (Kass 1975: 35). These right-wing criticisms of medicalization will be revisited in depth in later chapters. It is enough to note here that even in the early days of the critique of the growing dependence on professional-institutional health care, there was no clear-cut distinction along conventional political lines.

One problem with the medicalization thesis is that these writers have consistently underestimated patients' level of independence in the therapeutic relationship and the extent of critical attitudes towards the medical profession.

Throughout the 1970s the proponents of the medicalization thesis exaggerated the dominance of medical models of disease, ignoring the persistence of lay systems. This lack of awareness of the persistence of more traditional beliefs and practices can be seen clearly in Illich's discussion of cultural iatrogenesis, or the extent to which the popular consciousness had been reshaped by medical knowledge.

'Each culture', Illich observes, 'gives shape to a unique *Gestalt* of health and to a unique conformation of attitudes towards pain, disease, impairment, and death, each of which designates a class of that human performance that has traditionally been called the art of suffering' (Illich 1976: 69). In traditional cultures, he argues, healing serves to make 'pain tolerable, sickness or impairment understandable, and the shadow of death meaningful'. Most healing provides a way of 'consoling, caring, and comforting people while they heal, and most sick care a form of tolerance extended to the afflicted' (Illich 1976: 136–7). In traditional cultures, Illich reminds us, self-care is intrinsic to all spheres of the culture: 'health care is always a programme for eating, drinking, working, breathing, loving, politicking, exercising, singing, dreaming, warring, and suffering' (Illich 1976: 136). He argues that institutionalized health care undermines the continuation cultural patterns of self-care by discrediting traditional practices and preventing the emergence of new self-care cultures. The arts of suffering, healing and dying that traditional cultures taught each person

> are now claimed by technocracy as new areas of policy-making and are treated as malfunctions from which populations ought to be institutionally relieved. The goals of metropolitan medical civilization are thus in opposition to every single cultural health programme they encounter in the process of progressive colonization.
>
> (Illich 1976: 138)

Now, he believes, we only have a few remnants of peasant language in Western cultures to remind us of pre-medical understandings of illness (Illich 1976: 176). As I have discussed above, this is simply not the case. Patients are immersed in non-medical understandings and practices, and for doctors the problem of translating between medical and lay knowledges is part of their everyday work.

According to Illich, medicine pacifies its patients, who are no longer able to care for themselves or for their environment. In order to sustain this historical argument, Illich constructs an image of a past in which health care was provided intimately and passionately, and in which, although often powerless over their own body state, people had access to a culturally produced art of suffering which allowed them to experience their own body states as a private affair which only they could really know. In his description of pre-medicalized self-care, Illich focuses on 'the art of suffering', which, regardless of the sophistication of curative health-care systems, is an inescapable part of life. Modern medicine, instead of helping people to deal with their suffering on an interpersonal and spiritual level, represses such emotional and existential issues in favour of a doomed quest for a cure for pain, transforming the sick person into 'a limp and mystified voyeur of his [*sic*] own treatment' (Illich 1976: 111). The more that people place their faith in medicine to overcome their suffering, the more they deprive themselves of the coping resources they need to deal with the inescapable frailty of their bodies.

Illich and the other critics of medicalization are describing a shift in the dominant form of the constitution of self-care practices, from the face-to-face to the professional-institutional level of integration. They overemphasize medicine's ability to reconstitute self-care practices and largely disregard the effects of more general social changes in the form of integration. Traditional forms of self-care were above all undermined by the broader processes of modernization such as urbanization, which eroded agrarian lifestyle practices, and by the reduction in transmission of oral cultures across the generations with the break-up of the extended family. Despite its colonizing mentality, as I have argued earlier, medicine did not generally concern itself with proactive self-care promotion – it had developed neither the expertise nor the means of communication required to disseminate comprehensive lifestyle advice to the general public.

Self-care as a solution to institutional dependence

In the wake of these critiques of institutional health care in the 1970s, many commentators on health issues saw the promotion of self-care as a means of overcoming the problems of professional dependency. Levin, Katz and Holst's book *Self-Care: Lay Initiatives in Health* (1979) was inspired by and based on an international symposium on 'The Role of the Individual in Health Care', held in Copenhagen in 1975. As far as the authors were aware, this was the first international gathering to consider the role of self-care in health. There was already widespread popular interest in self-care but this had so far had little impact on institutional health-care systems. The participants at Copenhagen were keen to redress the over-reliance on professionals and employ self-care as a resource in the health-care system. They follow in Illich's political path, with the Symposium believing that 'in contrast with previous strategies for change [...] developing lay self-care competence has a powerful potential for deprofessionalizing the health care system' (L. Levin *et al.* 1979: 27).

In 1975, another international symposium on 'The Limits of Medicine', held in Switzerland, considered similar themes. In closing that conference, Dr Alex Comfort observed that self-care was becoming a major area of innovation in medical research and held the key to reversing what were seen as the negative consequences of medicalization. Comfort noted optimistically:

> If we look at medicine in general, I think it has already trended away from its past commodity and technology image by the logic of its research future. Some of its most promising innovations in medical technique already involve active patient self-help in a social setting. [...] This, if we can develop it, promises a technology of medical self-control which has the

potential for substituting almost wholly for drugs, in the management of conditions such as epilepsy, [...] hypertension and anxiety.

(cited in L. Levin *et al.* 1979: 2–3)

Most of those promoting anti-institutional self-care were liberal sociologists of health and public health practitioners who were sympathetic with Zola and Illich's critiques and were in search of practical measures to revitalize health-care systems which were under increasing public scrutiny. Self-care provided an inspiring range of possibilities, and encouraging personal responsibility seemed to allow the health-care system to work alongside contemporary cultural movements, which were obviously heading in this direction. Many advocates of self-care believed they were witnessing the emergence of a new social movement. When Ilona Kickbusch (later to become WHO director of health promotion) and Stephen Hatch described the popularity of self-care, they appeared to be reporting on an orchestrated campaign being waged by motivated activists: 'already both within and between countries the proponents are building networks of support to add impetus for the reinterpretation of the role of lay people in health' (Kickbush and Hatch 1983: 1). There appeared to be an alignment of various interests and early signs that the disparate manifestations of self-care in health would coalesce into a full-blown social movement (L. Levin *et al.* 1979: 35).

Adding weight to these calls was the fact that in the 1970s the role of the patient in shaping the illness experience and outcome had become readily apparent. To summarize the discussion above, a number of features of the active patient had become obvious: the decision to consult a professional is made by the patient, and is often the result of consultation with close family and friends; a large proportion of health care takes place without seeking medical advice; treatment decisions are often heavily influenced by the patient; the level of patient compliance with professionals is highly variable; patients evaluate the efficacy and outcomes of professional care (L. Levin *et al.* 1979: 14–15). Kickbusch and Hatch saw the 'discovery' of the self-active patient as a revolutionary development in the organization of health-care systems:

At the beginning of the 1980s it is becoming increasingly clear that health is not just something between doctors and patients: people are not merely consumers of health care, they pursue health and provide health care themselves through a broad range of activities that until recently have escaped the interest of policy makers, professionals and researchers. We are witness to a reorientation in health care provision which might prove as fundamental in the long run as the rise of the medical profession 150 years ago.

(Kickbusch and Hatch 1983: 1)

The demedicalization fallacy

Typical of the anti-institutional politics of self-care promotion is McEwen, Martin and Wilkins' call for 'an active involvement by the individual in all aspects of his or her own health care rather than the traditional passive role normally associated with being a patient' (McEwen *et al*. 1983: 2). They advocate 'improving the health care competence of lay people' in an effort to put a brake on cost escalation, increased demand for medical services, and increasing dependency on professional care. The active participation they propose manifests itself on two levels: 'a process of substitution and/or complementation whereby tasks normally thought to fall within the medical or professional sphere are taken on by the individual ("demedicalization" or "deprofessionalization")'; and 'the democratization of social policy and health care provision, where greater public accountability could be achieved through self-care, by empowering consumers in relation to service providers' (McEwen *et al*. 1983: 2).

These goals sound very appealing. People are to be freed from their reliance on professionals, allowing for both more autonomous self-care actions and the democratization of the health-care system as empowered consumers challenge professional authority over decision-making. The serious flaw in this type of anti-institutional politics is that it ignores the fact that the encouragement of self-care actually draws the health-care system deeper into the private life of the person and facilitates an expansion of professional power in new realms of life which were not previously of interest to the system. McEwen, Martin and Wilkins seem to acknowledge this at times, observing that

> a different outlook on education is required: one which encourages people, from a basis of knowledge, to choose between different paths of action, to make decisions and participate meaningfully in both their own health and in the provision of health and related services.
>
> (McEwen *et al*. 1983: 140)

That is, educators must provide the encouragement and the knowledge on which decisions will be based. Rather than a shift in power from the expert to the lay, what is occurring here is a reorientation in the nature of health expertise, from a form of expertise which pacifies the subject to one which activates the subject.

In a very literal use of the 'expansionary' understanding of the rise of self-care, Illich (1976) theorizes the relationship between self-care and professional care as a zero-sum equation. The only way self-care can expand is for a contraction of professional care to occur:

> The level of public health corresponds to the degree to which the means and responsibility for coping with an illness are distributed among the total population. This ability to cope can be enhanced but never replaced by medical intervention or by the hygienic characteristics of the environment.

That society which can reduce professional intervention to the minimum will provide the best conditions for health.

(Illich 1976: 274)

While hesitantly supporting measures such as nationalization of health-care systems, support for alternative therapies, consumer involvement in planning, and increased emphasis on prevention, Illich's overall attitude seems to be that institutional actors should disengage from health care as much as possible and let people fend for themselves. One measure that illustrates the naïveté of many of Illich's plans for self-reliance is his stance on dangerous personal practices. 'Instead of restricting access to addictive, dangerous, or useless drugs and procedures', he proposes that legislation should 'shift the full burden of their responsible use onto the sick person and his next of kin' (Illich 1976: 273–4). Despite the rhetoric of concentrating on the social causes of illness and of health behaviour, when it comes to countering medicalization, Illich sounds very much like conservative proponents of individual responsibility. The conservative commentator Leon Kass also made a similar call for health-care professionals to disengage from self-care. Paradoxically, he encourages the state to engage in broad lifestyle-oriented health promotion, which should 'increase personal responsibility for health' (Kass 1975: 37). He, like Illich, argues that there is a moral obligation on individuals to lead a healthy life, and goes on to argue that it is dangerous for governments to take advantage of this obligation by overemphasizing health concerns over other social goods, especially in cases where health may come in conflict with industrial activity or personal freedoms. But while conservative commentators have openly detailed their moral framework and how they think the state should act, Illich seems to just want to leave people alone to make their own decisions. He seems not to understand that contemporary self-care practices are being shaped more powerfully than ever before and has no interest in the rapidly expanding field of self-care promotion.

In 1985, Illich reflected on his earlier work on health and medicalization, expressing his amazement at the extent of the popular pursuit of the healthy body. The level of interest in non-medical health care had increased dramatically while the medical profession was being criticized openly. His call for the reduction of the power of the medical profession had been realized but he had failed to foresee the emergence of 'a curious mixture of opinionated and detailed self-care practices joined to a naïve enthusiasm for sophisticated technology' which had greatly undermined the personal attention offered by medical practitioners (Illich 1992: 212). Illich was able to see the medical colonization of health care clearly enough; however, he missed the current phase of the colonization of self-care, which was being led not by medicine but by new actors.

When they called for a return to 'autonomous' self-care, the critics of medicalization, concerned at the extent to which medicine undermined patients' capacities to care for themselves and increased their reliance on professionals, had no idea that self-care practices would be so thoroughly shaped by their producers and that the resulting autonomy would be linked to the freedom to consume the range of commodified self-care advice and practices provided within the market.

In the end, the call to empower individuals by limiting the power of health-care institutions was doomed. By the early 1980s the extent to which self-care practices had been thoroughly reconstituted by more abstract forms of self-care promotion had become apparent. The desire for freedom from the constraints imposed by institutionalized forms of care was channelled into consumer freedom in the expanded health-care market. The nostalgia for more concrete self-care practices, which had motivated the critique of the medicalization of life, had been taken up by the natural health movement, which provided people with mountains of advice about how to get back to nature. But there was no going back.

6   The nagging state

> The autonomous individual who is enabled to make better decisions in his or her own interest can improve health and moderate costs. [...] Health policies that encourage persons to place a higher value on health and that provide them with the tools necessary to take greater charge of their own health are required
>
> J.F. Fries *et al.*, 'Beyond health promotion' (1998: 77, 81)

The popular and academic interest in self-care in the 1970s was paralleled in public health policy by widespread calls for a new approach to public health. Public health was given new support by advocates of social medicine who argued in the 1960s and 1970s that clinical medical practice had not been the major factor in health status improvements in modern societies, as will be discussed in the following chapter. The greater effectiveness of 'social medicine' over clinical medicine in improving the health of whole populations was reaffirmed but the forms of public health that were being advocated were rather different from their nineteenth -century predecessors. What was new was, firstly, that social research throughout the previous decade had shown that self-care was a much more important determinant of well-being than professional care, which led to an extensive interest in the role of the individual in health care. Secondly, public health practitioners were aware of the recent interest in self-care evident in the popularity of self-help books, diets, exercise fads, self-help groups and alternative therapies. While on a popular level the natural health movement advised eating organic fruit and vegetables, de-stressing with yoga and meditation, and so on, governments began warning their citizens not to smoke and promoted the benefits of regular exercise. Many of the major health concerns of the period, particularly cancer and heart disease, had been shown to be influenced by self-care practices and came to be seen as 'lifestyle' diseases.

The problem the state had to face, arising from the perception that modern life is inherently harmful, was the dramatic complexification and extension of the domain of health care. This was in effect the second wave of the 'socialization' of health. At the beginning of the industrial era it became clear that the health of urban populations was as much a product of the social conditions in which people lived as it was due to natural causes. Late in the twentieth century the known social determinants of health became much more extensive (summed up in the cliché that 'everything gives you cancer'). Because of the apparent health consequences involved in every aspect of one's life, the management of health by the state became a much more difficult endeavour. A common argument found within much recent public health literature is that health promotion policies require a 'holistic' approach, or what in government is called 'intersectoral collaboration' or a 'whole of government approach'. The Australian National Health Strategy's review of health promotion programmes, for example, explained that 'health has become too complicated to be left to health ministers, departments and professionals', and called for engagement with other dimensions of life, including the spheres of business, agriculture, education and transport (National Health Strategy 1993: 13).

The state responded to the first stage in the socialization of health largely through legislative action, and the political debates that ensued were typically carried out within a liberal framework, requiring constant justification of the need for state intervention in light of its capacity to restrict individual freedom. In the 1970s, because of the awareness of self-care and the political climate of the times, most of the proposals for the new public health lay in new forms of intervention. From the 1970s onwards, public health became much more interdisciplinary, drawing on the social sciences, including sociology and social work, and drawing in nurses, educators, planners, demographers and accountants. Often the health needs of the population were still determined epidemiologically, but the technologies with which to facilitate the behavioural and social engineering necessary to improve health were provided by disciplines with very different outlooks to medicine. This is not the place to delve into the inter-professional politics that ensued, but what is important to note is that the comparatively cosy relationship between medicine and the state which characterized public health in earlier eras was upset by the entry of these new groups of workers and new opportunities for state action with which medicine was unfamiliar.

Modern governments have long tried to improve the health of their citizens in various ways, but since the 1970s they have increasingly done this through informational campaigns aimed at changing opinions and behaviour. It was only in the late 1970s and early 1980s that governments in late capitalist societies set about promoting self-care practices in a systematic way. Until this time the popular interest in self-care had been quite distinct from public health policies (L. Levin *et al.* 1979: 4). Since the 1970s, however, there has been a vast increase in the effort the state makes to tell its citizens how to behave, making governments just one more source of self-care advice. To put it very simply, there are basically four ways in which the state can attempt to improve the health of its population. They can support biomedical research, provide or otherwise ensure access to health care, ameliorate health hazards in the physical and social environment, and encourage individuals to lead more healthy lifestyles (Leichter 1991).

Public health is concerned with the latter two forms of state intervention, and in this chapter I will chart the way in which public health has broadened from the third of these, a concern with environment, to the fourth, a concern with lifestyles. The central terms of public health are essentially contested and form the basis of incessant and sometimes fierce debates among practitioners and policy makers, so a degree of slipperiness in descriptions of rival approaches is inevitable. Not wanting to delve into these debates overly, I will follow generally accepted usage and employ the terms 'lifestyle approach', 'health education' and 'behavioural modification approach' almost interchangeably (Beattie 1991).

The 'old' public health

There were two distinct systems of medical classification and management in operation in the nineteenth century – clinical medicine and public health. While clinical medicine was concerned with the separation of the normal and the abnormal, the physiological and the pathological, public health was centred on a notion of disease which focused on the relationship between the interior of the body and its physical environment, and particularly the movement of 'dirt' and other forms of contamination across this boundary (Armstrong 1988: 8–9). Public health comprised an alliance of science and the state, recommending and enforcing laws which regulated water quality, food hygiene in production and retailing, building codes, pest control, quarantine laws, vaccination and immunization campaigns, and so on (Roe 1984). Early public health developed as the state sought to respond to the health problems caused by the physical environment of the city. All cities required centralized management of the supply of water, the removal of sewage, the disposal of the dead, the removal of the dangerously criminal or insane, as well as the general maintenance of basic infrastructure such as roads which allows urban life to continue. The modern industrial city of nineteenth-century Europe, however, produced new problems. Rapid rates of urban growth caused the concentration of much larger populations into poor and overcrowded housing. New production methods, coal fires and inadequate amenities resulted in extensive pollution of air and waterways. Poor working conditions caused high rates of industrial accidents, and repetitive work and long hours took a heavy toll on manual workers' bodies (Engels 1973; Percival 1973).

Britain was one of the earliest urbanized nations, with the 1851 census reporting that for the first time just over half the population lived in cities with over 10,000 people, while by century's end this figure was 77 per cent (Leichter 1991: 35). Many of the early public health models which came to be used in the USA and Australia were first developed in Britain, making it a useful starting point in discussing subsequent developments in these countries. In Britain in the nineteenth century, the dominance of laissez-faire economics and liberal political philosophies held back state action to remedy the social problems caused by industrialization, which were disproportionately borne by the working class. It is interesting to note that in this political environment the use of state authority to improve living conditions occurred earlier in the field of public health than in other forms of welfare, such as education, labour laws, building regulations or financial assistance for the poor (Leichter 1991: 36). This was perhaps due to the fact that the epidemic diseases such as cholera, typhus and smallpox which struck the nation in waves were not confined to the poor. A major motivation for state involvement was the fear that contagious diseases caused by the unsanitary conditions of the working class could spread to the middle and upper classes (Turner 1991). National statistics of illness began to be recorded from 1837, and within a few years, after the smallpox epidemic of 1837–40, which resulted in 41,644 deaths, the first Vaccination Act (1840) was passed (although vaccination had been introduced to Britain in 1798). This Act provided free vaccination to anyone and was the first use of medicine by the state in Britain (Leichter 1991: 38–9).

There were two economic arguments in this period to support public health. The first was put forward in Edwin Chadwick's influential *Report on the Sanitary Condition of the Labouring Population of Great Britain* (1842), of which over 10,000 copies were circulated. Chadwick argued that poor living conditions often caused the death of breadwinners and drove people to destitution and the poor-houses, where they were a burden to ratepayers, or to hospitals, which were also funded by the wealthy. These costs could be reduced by providing more effective sanitation and better living conditions for the poor. The government responded to this report in 1848, passing the Public Health Act, which established a national authority to enforce and coordinate the range of public health measures in which the state was becoming involved.

The second argument centred on concerns that the poor health of the working class was undermining both the productive efficiency and the military strength of the nation. During the Crimean War (1853–6), concerns over the high rejection rates of working-class recruits led to warnings that 'unless the physical deterioration of the lower classes is stopped by bold sanitary reform [...] we shall soon have rifles but no men to shoulder them' (cited in Leichter 1991: 43). This issue resurfaced after the Boer War at the turn of the twentieth century with the publication in 1902 of an article by Major General Sir John Frederick Maurice entitled 'Where to get men?' The poor performance of the British army, he believed, was linked to the lack of physical stamina of working-class recruits, and he was concerned about difficulties in recruitment due to the poor health of those who applied. In the interests of maintaining a strong national defence, he warned that 'no nation was ever for any long time great and free, when the army it put in the field no longer represented its own virility and manhood' (Leichter 1991: 43). This led to a vigorous debate in the British press about causes of the 'physical deterioration' of the nation. Eugenicists worried aloud about the increase in the proportion of 'defective' or 'degenerate stock' in the population. In response the government established an Interdepartmental Committee on Physical Deterioration, which reported to Parliament in 1904. The committee found no evidence of physical deterioration in the population as a whole and instead focused on the poor health of the poorest of the working class, from whom the majority of recruits were drawn. As well as restating established views about the effects of overcrowding, pollution, poor sanitation and working conditions, the committee found that a lack of self-care amongst this group was responsible.

> In large classes of the community there has not been developed a desire for improvement commensurate with opportunities offered to them. Laziness, want of thrift, ignorance of household management, and particularly of the choice and preparation of food, filth, indifference to parental obligations, drunkenness, largely infect adults of both sexes, and press with terrible severity upon their children.
>
> (Leichter 1991: 44)

The committee recommended measures to tackle both the environmental and attitudinal problems it identified, emphasizing health education for the poor.

Despite the reluctance of nineteenth-century liberals to involve the state in the private affairs of its citizens, there was support for the state to uphold moral values, as is argued by the New Right today. So a fourth justification for public health intervention, alongside the fear of contagious disease, cost-effectiveness and national defence, was to curb the health problems associated with 'immoral' behaviour, particularly drunkenness and prostitution. From 1864 to 1886 laws were put in force which allowed for the forced examination and incarceration of female prostitutes who were believed to have venereal diseases. These laws also had a national defence orientation, initially applying to areas surrounding military installations, in order to decrease the incidence of venereal disease among soldiers. There was extensive opposition to these acts because, firstly, by regulating rather than outlawing prostitution, the state effectively supported the practice, and, secondly, these laws discriminated against women, depriving them of constitutional rights, while protecting the men who patronized prostitution (Leichter 1991: 47).

The environmental public health interventions during the nineteenth century dramatically improved living conditions by making the physical environment less harmful. David Armstrong (1983) identifies a shift early in the twentieth century to a model of public health which focused more squarely on the *social* spaces between bodies as the medium of transmission of disease rather than an older system of hygiene in which the boundaries between bodies and environment were policed. The 'new' public health which emerged around this attention to the social was inclined to treat the person as a more active participant in health care. As H.W. Hill stated in *The New Public Health* (1916), 'The old public health was concerned with the environment; the new is concerned with the individual' (cited in Armstrong 1988: 10). It is to this period that Armstrong traces the origins of public health's desire actively to shape individuals. The advocates of the new (social) hygiene pointed to its reliance on what a 1920 *British Medical Journal* editorial described as educated people 'willing and able to practice the way of health' (cited in Armstrong 1983: 11). The person was thus constructed not only as an active object of medicine (in that their own hygienic actions were seen to be important determinants of disease processes and therefore the domain of the medical gaze) but also as the active subject of their own care. In the nine-teenth century, Armstrong points out, only the public official had the ability to monitor and control the dangers posed by the environment. Now that the dangers were found to lie in the more intimate practices of persons themselves, the population had to be mobilized in new ways as the agents of their own care in order to ensure the application of public health knowledge (Armstrong 1988: 10). But while the authorities had at their disposal the means of surveillance, as Armstrong describes, they did not have the requisite means of persuasion needed to transform the lifestyles of the public. Apart from hygiene, they lacked persuasive evidence linking specific behaviours to specific diseases. Apart from schools, they lacked the means to convey such information to the public. So they concentrated for the time being on teaching personal hygiene in schools.

In the 1960s a number of advocates of social medicine argued that much of the improvement in the health status of populations in modern societies was due to social rather than medical advancements. One of the first of these was René Dubos (1960, 1968), whose 'ecological' view of health and illness had a consider-able influence on later critiques of medicine. Thomas McKeown, a British doctor and demographer, was particularly influential in arguing that improve-ments in living conditions, including nutrition, sanitation and water supply, had an enormous effect on health status (McKeown and Lowe 1974; McKeown 1976, 1979). He observed that while some aspects of lifestyle, most notably drug addiction and sexual promiscuity, had long been known to prejudice health, there were many self-care practices whose ill-effects had only recently become apparent, due both to increased incidence of these behaviours and to new tech-niques for linking self-care practices with long-term effects. For example, if the effects of smoking were manifested in thirty hours rather than thirty years, measures of control would have been introduced very quickly. The distant nature of smoking's effects hid it from scrutiny for a long time – both in terms of delayed effects and the probabilistic nature of its consequences rather than having definitely attributable consequences (McKeown and Lowe 1974: 125). Although these writers emphasized the importance of social context and envi-ronmental factors in influencing health, their work was taken up by advocates of self-care who argued that the individual is in a powerful position to be able to reduce the impact of such external factors on themselves through the modifica-tion of personal lifestyle. Despite being proposed in various forms repeatedly during most of the twentieth century, behavioural approaches to public health did not make a large impact on health-care systems until the 1970s.

Medicine's passive patients

After the Second World War, as medicine broadened its interest to encompass more 'normal' states such as childhood, old age, sexual functioning and psycho-logical states, it began to treat the healthy population as potentially at risk of illness. Epidemiological surveys of the distribution of symptoms and sociological insights into illness behaviour started to influence medical thinking, and the previously passive body came alive. Through the 1940s, psychological models made their way into medicine, encouraging an interest in the personality of the patient, and the earlier concerns with 'interrogating' the patient and avoiding 'defaulting' patients gradually came to be seen as problems of communication between a doctor and a complex psyche. However, it was not until the 1960s and 1970s that medical teaching manuals incorporated this concern with this more self-active and reflexive model of the subject to any extent (Armstrong 1983: 109). Although, as Armstrong notes, there was some discussion in medical circles about the desirability of a social approach to medical practice, 'social medicine' did not become established as a branch of medicine or begin to be introduced into medical courses until during the Second World War, and even then it was on a very small scale (Armstrong 1983: 38–41).

One of the defining texts of social medicine, McKeown and Lowe's *An Introduction to Social Medicine* (1966), devotes only ten of its 350 pages to the modification of personal behaviour, matter-of-factly discussing the dangers of smoking, alcohol, overeating and physical inactivity. This highlights how small the range of medically defined risk behaviours was in the 1960s, in comparison with the extensive links between behaviour and disease which have been suggested since, and in relation to these behaviours, self-care still seems to have had a minor role (McKeown and Lowe 1974: 117–26). This would appear to indicate that proponents of social medicine had a broader view of the social than simply individual lifestyles. However, there was just as little interest in self-care in other branches of medical practice in the period. A study of doctors in Los Angeles in the late 1970s found that a majority expressed negative attitudes to self-care. The authors concluded that the overall opinion of the medical practitioners they studied was that self-care 'would not reduce visits to the doctor, may create more harm than good, and that people cannot learn to take care of themselves adequately' (Linn and Lewis 1977: 189). The attitude of the medical profession seemed to be that 'a little knowledge is a dangerous thing' and that patients were likely to be confused or become anxious. Popular self-help books of the 1970s encouraged patients actively to question their doctor and to 'shop around' for other opinions – practices which were sure to annoy and undermine the authority of the professional in the medical encounter. In light of such attitudes from self-help advocates, it is understandable that doctors often saw the promotion of active health-seeking behaviour as a threat to their need to obtain patient compliance with their treatment decisions (L. Levin *et al.* 1979: 45). Indeed, although, more recently, most health-care professionals have been slowly embracing the use of some self-help groups and patient information materials under professional supervision, especially in treating behavioural conditions (Cooper *et al.* 1994), they are still very sceptical of much self-help literature and have little knowledge of appropriate self-care resources to suggest to their patients (Rosen 1987, 1994).

The transformation of health education

Up until the 1970s, health education had generally consisted of providing information to patients, either to teach them to act in a specified manner, or to elicit greater compliance with professionals' instructions. Health professionals were custodians of a body of expert knowledge which could be revealed strategically to the patient when it would prove helpful in treatment. The knowledge held by patients and other lay people was generally ignored by the practitioner, and when this knowledge conflicted with medical opinion, it was thought that providing authoritative scientific information would overcome potential problems with compliance (Ritchie 1991). The means by which the provision of information would lead to compliance was described by Becker's Health Belief Model. Compliant behaviour was seen to be determined by the patient or group's level of knowledge about their susceptibility to the condition, the severity of the condition, and steps which could be taken to minimize harm (Becker 1974). In response to evaluations which showed this type of health education to be not as effective as its practitioners had hoped, in the late 1960s many health educators began to diversify the means by which they delivered information, believing that with better means of presentation, greater retention and hence increased behavioural change would eventuate. A practising health educator at this time describes the physical demands which were made on educators in an effort to get the message across:

> Whereas in the previous era all that was needed was a reliable watch to be able to ascertain that the available time was filled with appropriate input, now access to all manner of audio-visual aids was essential. Films, projectors, screens, audio-cassette players, pamphlets, leaflets, posters, booklets all became part of the regular health education armamentarium, not to mention simulated body parts and complicated demonstration kits all aiming to reinforce verbal explanations.
>
> (Ritchie 1991: 158)

The mass media and advertising techniques were also being tapped in health promotion. While early evaluation of television advertising by itself yielded disappointing results, the combination of broad messages in the electronic media with professional contact and more closely targeted information seemed to work well (Rissel 1991). The media through which information was channelled had diversified, but the nature of the message, Ritchie (1991) argues, had not changed dramatically. Up to the 1980s, most health education was heavily influenced by American behaviourist psychology and had assumed that simply providing information (in the right way) was all that was needed to change behaviour. The information conveyed, regardless of the medium, still tended to be medical knowledge, presented by 'talking heads' in medical language involving little engagement with lay concepts of health and illness causation or with the everyday language of those who were being targeted.

The most extensive promotion of self-care by the state has been carried out within health education. This takes the form of 'primary' health education, which involves providing preventive information and advice to the public. ('Secondary' health education deals with the provision of what I am calling reactive self-care advice to those who are exhibiting symptoms, and 'tertiary' health education is directed at those who are living with a chronic condition.)

Within primary health education in recent decades there has been a gradual shift away from behaviourist models of education and behaviour modification to models which stress the importance of subjective processes in engaging with the information provided, interpreting it and making it meaningful. This shift parallels a similar move in the 1980s in literary theory with the popularity of post-structuralist and reader-response theories which viewed reading (in its broadest sense) as an active process which is never completely determined by authorial intent. In health education, as in education more generally, acknowledging the recipient of messages as an active interpreting agent led to educational models which attempted to use the subject's interpretive capacities to improve techniques of behavioural modification. Green *et al.* state that 'the evidence that the durability of cognitive and behavioral changes is proportional to the degree of active rather than passive participation of the learner is overwhelming' (Green *et al.* 1980: 8). The passive object of health information was now being seen in a new light, as a necessarily active participant in the learning and change process. To a limited extent, health education embraced the open text by de-emphasizing the authority of expert knowledge and pointing to the advantages of providing the opportunity for those being taught to add meaning to the information by interacting to shape its content. Ritchie describes this as having a positive impact on the self-worth of health educational professionals, who were

> at last able to feel that they had something of value to give their community members. The frustration of putting a lot of work into educational programs that were relatively fruitless gave way to a realization that people could and would change, but on their own terms.
>
> (Ritchie 1991: 159)

Through working with the individual's expressed understandings as the basis upon which to build expert knowledge, and using the reflexivity of the subject as a strategy to elicit behavioural change, health educators gained a sense of satisfaction from seeing individuals 'becoming more self-reliant and self-responsible for their own health, and were ready to praise those whose health had improved through their own actions' (Ritchie 1991: 159). Reflecting this shift, the WHO now defines health education more broadly than the provision of information, to encompass fostering self-care motivation, skills and confidence: 'Health education comprises consciously constructed opportunities for learning involving some form of communication designed to improve health literacy, including improving knowledge, and developing life skills which are conducive to individual and community health' (Nutbeam 1998: 4). Health education now uses more sophisticated communication techniques rather than the straightforward presentation of health facts. The earlier emphasis on health knowledge as expressed in the 'health beliefs' model of health education has been expanded to include the cultivation of the audience's life skills and motivation to change their behaviour.

One area in which the state has become most noticeably involved in fostering the reflexive self-care of individuals is in the education system. Physical education began in British schools early in the twentieth century with the application of military training techniques, which were later tailored specifically for school environments. Rather than aiming to improve the physical fitness of students as an end in itself, the intention of the Board of Education, as stated in 1909, was that through repetitive drill training 'the child unconsciously acquires habits of discipline and order, and learns to respond cheerfully and promptly to the word of command' (cited in Armstrong 1988: 11–12). Later this sentiment is repeated by the Board in 1928, which insists that its object is not merely health in a physical sense but the broader character of the child. The Board writes, 'Physical fitness should not be advocated by the teacher as an end in itself, but as a means to promote the mental and moral health and character of the child.' Although this form of physical education was intended to have a variety of effects – moral, intellectual and physiological – the education was thoroughly pacifying in the sense that it did not require the students to be self-directed or proactive in their self-care. Students were subjected to repetitive exercises in military fashion because in the opinion of the British Board of Education, as stated in their 1909 syllabus of physical training for schools, 'undirected indiscriminate exercise cannot take the place of a scientific system of training' (cited in Armstrong 1988: 35).

Today, health education in schools is extensive, comprising units such as physical education, home economics (nutrition, cooking), human development, personal development, and so on. Increasingly the types of health problems being identified require an education that deals not only with the body and health maintenance behaviour but also with issues of self-identity, self-image and self-esteem. A text for early secondary school students produced by the South Australian Education Department is typical in its content. Entitled *Body Owner's Manual for Secondary Students and Their Parents*, as well as sections on anatomy, physiology, smoking, alcohol and the traditional concerns of public health, much of the text is directed to self-evaluation and to heightening self-care by the bodies' owners. Chapter headings include 'Lifestyle can be a health hazard', 'You've got to work on your health right now', 'Your good health depends on you' and 'Taking control' (Coonan *et al.* 1986). Another popular secondary school text (for later year students in this case, and much more comprehensive) begins with a chapter entitled 'Health, personal identity and relationships' (including a section on 'Establishing a personal identity') which sets the rest of the book's discussion of health firmly within a context of the total management of one's life (Davy 1994). Being healthy requires as a first step the competent management of one's personality, in order to provide a stable ontological platform from which the person can care for their own well-being. While schools have always trained children, for the school system actively to heighten the reflexive awareness of children through teaching the application of behavioural sciences significantly changes the nature of education and the school's involvement in the constitution of self-identity.

Through the 'interpellation' (Althusser 1977) of the self-active subject via the classroom, advertising and public education, the state both participates in and responds to the detraditionalization of more culturally embedded practices of the self. While at the same time exerting more control over the individual, these developments have, in one sense, 'handed back' responsibility to the individual, so that health is now seen more than ever as one's personal responsibility. And similarly, the emotional, economic and spiritual well-being of the person has become reconceptualized as the responsibility of the self-active subject who is both empowered to care for themselves and is liable to be blamed if they do not care for themselves appropriately.

Lifestyle modification in public health

In practice, the focus of lifestyle approaches is usually determined by behavioural epidemiology, that is, through a medical understanding of the relationship between specific diseases and 'risk' behaviours, which are treated as discrete and independently modifiable practices. This form of health promotion aims to provide individuals with the motivation, knowledge and skills needed to prevent the onset of disease. The objective of public self-care promotion is the modification of an individual's 'lifestyle', a term which has taken on an atomistic meaning as the sum of an individual's personal habits (Coreil *et al.* 1985).

In the 1970s, health promotion advocates began to receive considerable support from the Right, who saw self-care advice as one means of reducing the state's health-care costs by shifting the burden of responsibility onto individuals. American Victor Fuchs' influential overview of health economics, *Who Shall Live?* (1974), emphasized the part that lifestyle plays in determining health status. He states that the notion of a 'right to health' prominent in contemporary literature suggests that society has a store of health which it distributes to the population. If health is held to be in short supply or unequitably distributed, there is a tendency to see this as a result of inefficient government, a profit-driven health-care system or a self-interested medical profession. These critiques, he says, vastly underestimate the self-inflicted nature of much illness. While discussions of lifestyle and health make up only a small part of Fuchs' book, the belief that much greater health gain can be achieved through attitudinal and behavioural change formed a major part of his approach to resolving some of the pressing issues in health economics. 'The greatest potential for improving the health of the American people', he concluded, 'is to be found in what they do and don't do for themselves' (Fuchs 1974: 54–5).

Throughout the late 1970s and 1980s, against a backdrop of fiscal crisis and an emergent New Right, health economists became interested in epidemiological research, which had suggested that medicine's impact on the long-term changes in the health status of populations was not as great as the profession had claimed. Arguments were mounted as to the economic benefits that could be gained by employing more efficient disease-preventive measures rather than further increasing spending on acute care services. In this political context, self-care was, from the early days of its promotion, seen as a means of cost containment in health care. Liberal writers concerned with patient 'empowerment' will strategically employ arguments pointing to cost savings to support their case, despite being uneasy when health economists justify funding cuts to institutional services in the same way. Likewise those on the Right are inclined to use the rhetoric of personal empowerment and individual responsibility to support cost-cutting measures inspired by a belief in the necessity of a minimal role for the state.

An influential Canadian government working paper, officially entitled *A New Perspective on the Health of Canadians* but widely referred to as the Lalonde report after its author, provided a seminal expression of this lifestyle modification approach at the level of policy proposals (Lalonde 1974). The major causes of mortality and 'premature' morbidity (including motor-vehicle accidents, ischaemic heart disease, respiratory diseases, lung cancer and suicide) are attributable primarily to risks stemming from both lifestyle and environmental factors, Lalonde argued. The 'new perspective' effectively broadened the scope of health policy by placing environmental health and lifestyle modification on a par with the traditional fields of health-care service provision.

The following year, in 1975, a sub-committee of the British House of Commons Expenditure Committee was set the task of examining the problem of increasing health costs. The committee reported that it was 'particularly interested in the prevalence of disease precipitated by the individual's habits [...] sometimes described to us as "disease of civilization" or "self-induced disease" ', concluding that 'we have been convinced by our enquiry that substantial human and financial resources would be saved if greater emphasis were placed on prevention' (United Kingdom Expenditure Committee 1977: xvi). Whereas environmental public health had been successful in the past, 'today, the greatest scope for further progress would seem to lie in seeking to modify attitudes and behaviour in relation to health' (10). While the government did not support banning tobacco advertising, placing stronger messages on cigarette packets, banning cigarette machines in premises available to minors, and a number of other measures recommended by the committee, it did implement the health education proposals that had been called for. Even within the Labour Party there was a predilection for behavioural over structural or regulative change, which the committee's report made explicit by drawing attention to the self-inflicted nature of many illnesses. 'Much ill health in Britain today', the report states, 'arises from over-indulgence and unwise behaviour. Not surprisingly, the greatest potential and perhaps the greatest problem for preventive medicine now lies in changing behaviour and attitudes to health' (10).

The committee's report coincided with a discussion document prepared by the Department of Health and Social Security (1976) entitled *Prevention and*

Health: Everybody's Business. While acknowledging that state action was important, it stated that,

> To a large extent though, it is clear that the weight of responsibility for his [sic] own health lies on the shoulders of the individual himself. The smoking related diseases, alcoholism and other drug dependencies, obesity and its consequences, and the sexually transmitted diseases are among the preventable problems of our time and in relation to all of these the individual must choose for himself.
>
> (38)

Within the American health administration in the late 1970s, it was understood that health promotion priorities generated according to such bureaucratic logics and administered through technocratic means had to be imposed from above by the state. Personal responsibility was seen as the key to 'effective and cost-effective health', but conservative policy-makers were aware that the type of personal responsibility they wanted to see was, according to an adviser to the US Department of Health, Education and Welfare, 'not generated spontaneously among population groups. It is the result of motivation created by leadership which is charismatic, knowledgeable and convinced that personal responsibility for health is a major solution to a major problem' (Watkin 1978: 3). In such accounts, the privatization of responsibility for health is portrayed as a simple economic necessity, which was later allied with a New Right personal empowerment rhetoric in the following years under the Reagan administration. The argument that expanding professional interest in self-care would reduce health-care costs is based on two expectations: that more knowledgeable actors will be more discriminating in their usage of professional services; and that expertly informed health maintenance behaviour will result in lower rates of preventable illness, thereby reducing demand for professional services. One study of the economic effects of self-care on professional services estimated that if 2 per cent of over-the-counter drug consumers opted to visit health-care practitioners instead of self-medicating, the number of patient visits to primary care practitioners would rise by 62 per cent (Rottenberg 1980). Levin, Katz and Holst argue that investments in self-care promotion may be more efficient because 'skills possessed by consumers are immediately available as productive output, self-adjusting and discriminately applied according to self-observed effectiveness' (L. Levin *et al.* 1979: 26).

The 1979 United States Surgeon General's Report drew a clear distinction between older disease prevention models of public health and health promotion. 'Disease prevention begins with a threat to health – a disease or environmental hazard – and seeks to protect as many people as possible from the harmful consequences of that threat', whereas 'health promotion begins with people who are basically healthy and seeks the development of community and individual measures which can help them to develop lifestyles that can maintain and enhance the state of well-being' (United States Department of Health,

Education and Welfare 1979: 119). The reason identified, which necessitates this intervention, is the pathogenic nature of everyday life and intimate acts:

> Personal habits play critical roles in the development of many serious diseases and in injuries from violence and automobile accidents. Many of today's most pressing health problems are related to excess smoking, drinking, faulty nutrition, overuse of medication, fast driving, and relentless pressure to achieve.
>
> (United States Department of Health, Education and Welfare 1979: 119)

This points to the power that the state must wield through self-care promotion if it is to curb 'excess'. There is a clear normative dimension in the state's attempts to impose the healthy lifestyle on its citizens, regardless of the means employed (Rosenstock 1990). However, throughout the health promotion literature the power being exercised through the imposition of a set of values is largely ignored in favour of a technocratic rationality directed at 'objective' risks that leaves cultural values unexamined. Health promotion, this report says, consists of 'activities which individuals and communities can use to promote healthy lifestyles' (United States Department of Health, Education and Welfare 1979: 81). Through the language of active participation and autonomous action, the issue of whose version of the lifestyle is being imposed on whom is consistently set aside. Health promotion, according to its advocates, 'works with people, not on them', mobilizing the self-care capacities of an active population (S. Brown and Szoke 1988: 37). Seedhouse (1997) refers to this as health promotion's outsider problem, arguing that the discipline does not have an adequate political or philosophical framework for dealing with values which do not accord with its own, such as someone who is determined to live 'to excess' even though they are aware of the health consequences of such actions.

The then United States Secretary for Health, Education and Welfare, Joseph Califano, writing in the foreword to the 1979 Surgeon General's report, stressed that these policies were being promulgated not only in the interests of those whose self-care was to be improved, but on behalf of the society as a whole. Califano bluntly warned the American public to take more care of themselves: 'We are killing ourselves by our own careless habits. [...] You the individual can do more for your own health and well-being than any doctor, any hospital, any drug, any exotic medical device' (United States Department of Health, Education and Welfare 1979: viii). He pointed to an obligation on the individual to engage in self-care in the collective interest, stating that 'indulgence in "private" excesses has results that are far from private. Public expenditures for health care that consume eleven cents for every federal tax dollar are only one of those results' (United States Department of Health, Education and Welfare 1979: ix). This public interest argument gives the state the right to intervene to shape personal behaviour even when the person whose health is in question seems to have little interest in such self-care. During this period, John Knowles, former president of the Rockefeller Foundation, entered the debate, stating that 'the cost of sloth, gluttony, alcoholic intemperance, reckless driving, sexual frenzy and smoking have now become a national not an individual responsibility. One man's or woman's freedom in health is now another man's shackles in taxes and insurance premiums' (cited in Crawford 1979: 255).

The Surgeon General's report went on to estimate that 50 per cent of mortality was due to unhealthy behaviour or lifestyle, 20 per cent to environmental factors, 20 per cent to human biology, and 10 per cent to deficiencies in the health-care system. Given the meaninglessness of these numbers, this crude attempt to reduce mortality to simple mono-causal agents can only be read as a rhetorical device in support of a policy orientation, since there is no way that, even in the case of one death, the relative weight of these intrinsically inter-related factors can be determined, let alone at the population level. State action is legitimated by the argument that health-care costs are a burden on the society; therefore individuals have a responsibility not to engage in practices which may increase their reliance on health-care services.

In 1980, the US Public Health Service published *Promoting Health/Preventing Disease: Objectives for the Nation*, which couched health promotion in the context of budgetary restraint. Its introduction stated: 'At a time in the Nation's history when budgets become tighter, legislators, public officials and governing boards of industry, foundations, universities and voluntary agencies are beginning to re-examine their traditional bases for allocating their limited health-related resources' (United States Department of Health and Human Services 1980: vii). The report put forward 226 objectives which were to be reached by 1990. Some of these were met, such as reducing the number of motor-vehicle injuries and deaths, reducing the rate of smoking and alcohol consumption, while some were not, such as reducing the number of adults overweight, or increasing the number who exercise regularly (Leichter 1991). The point is that each of these social changes was deemed necessary because of the cost it imposed on the health-care system. These economic arguments will be discussed in more detail below.

In Australia similar sentiments were expressed in the Commonwealth Health Department's report *Health Promotion in Australia* (Davidson *et al.* 1979). This did, however, acknowledge the difficulty in changing health behaviour and was critical of 'the prevailing orthodoxy' in public health policy which assumes that 'people are free to choose certain health-related behaviours or lifestyles. However, this narrow sense of "choice" fails to account for the adaptive value of behaviour to the life-situation of the individual' (11–12). The report described this approach as 'victim-blaming', and called for greater governmental effort in 'the alteration of constraints on health that are beyond the control of individuals' (13). In the end, however, it argued that in many cases individual behaviour is easier to change than structural determinants of health status, and, given the impediments to significant structural change, policies which focus on individual choice are called for:

> Positive changes in national health status are unlikely to occur without fundamental and substantial changes in social and economic organization.

[...] What is the practising health promoter to do while waiting for society to realize that it cannot afford premature coronary artery disease? It is here that the micro or individual approach presents itself as a practical solution. [...] Given that broad and sweeping social change conducive to improved community health is unlikely, national health promotion must concentrate on the most effective ways of motivating changes in those areas where individual choice finally determines behaviour.

(13–14)

Governments have in this way willingly participated in the individualization of risk management in an effort to depoliticize socially produced risks by focusing on individual choices rather than the social contexts which shape such behaviours. Even when the broader determinants of health are acknowledged, self-care practices are seen to be the most effective means of state intervention to improve health.

Even if heightened health consciousness did lead to decreased use of medical services, health-related spending has dramatically increased in other areas. Greater interest in exercise will fuel demand in the fitness industry, leading to increased spending on sporting equipment, gym memberships, and so on. Broader knowledge of the diversity of available services may lead to greater utilization of physiotherapists, naturopaths, masseurs, and so on, and expert self-care advice itself comes at a price, whether through books, courses or from personal trainers. When economic arguments for self-care promotion are discussed, the very different interests of institutional actors are rarely acknowledged. Most who point to the cost-effectiveness of self-care do not acknowledge that while purchasers of health care (whether individuals, families, the state or health insurance companies) have an interest in cost containment, providers of care, on the other hand (including providers of self-care), generally have an interest in economic expansion through either greater quantity or unit cost of services. The groups benefiting economically from tapping into self-care include the fitness industry, manufacturers of health foods, sporting goods and lay health-care products, and alternative and allied health-care professions. Health insurance companies and the state are likely to benefit from the shifting of costs from a form of health care they traditionally subsidize – medicine and hospital services – to services traditionally funded by the patient through fee-for-service. For the medical profession, increased encouragement of self-care and heightened health consciousness involves the possibility of losing both sole authority over their patients and their professional dominance over the swelling field of health care.

During the late 1970s and late 1980s, the Left's stronghold was in the community health movement, and in particular in local health centres, often catering to poor or marginalized groups. A stark political division developed within public health between those with a communitarian focus, who work to empower groups and communities to care for their own health, and those who focus on personal lifestyle change. Conflict between these two approaches to self-care is widespread within public health, and while a variety of strategies are employed to address any specific public health issue, the relative weight (and funding) accorded to each approach constitutes an ongoing source of disagreement and political debate.

Many on the Left see self-care approaches in health as nothing more than a convenient rationale used by the New Right to slash welfare spending, and so have generally focused on the economic motivations for such approaches. The New Right's philosophy of empowering individuals through a more thorough integration into the market obviously goes hand in hand with tax-cuts for the wealthy and reductions in welfare spending (Sawicky 1992). In the 1970s, it was routinely argued that the burgeoning welfare state, of which health care comprises a substantial proportion, could be brought under control by passing some of the increasing costs back to consumers. The Left pointed out that the assertion of individual responsibility for health through self-care promotion has been used to justify the removal of funds from public health-care systems in favour of individualized consumer advice and self-insurance (Salmon 1984; Coward 1989). During the 1980s in the United States this connection was made explicit as social welfare agencies were forced to experiment with self-help approaches to service delivery after massive budget cuts (Turem and Born 1983).

During the 1980s, there was widespread criticism of lifestyle approaches to public health especially in the sociology of health and social medicine. The failure of lifestyle health promotion to deal adequately with the sociocultural context of behaviour came to be seen a major weakness. While the lifestyle approach grew out of a scholarly tradition which emphasized social context and cultural meanings, the application of lifestyle health promotion largely ignored systemic influences, instead focusing almost exclusively upon individual responsibility (Coreil and Levin 1984; Coreil *et al.* 1985). Robert Crawford (1977, 1979, 1980) led the critique of the victim-blaming tendencies of lifestyle health promotion. He argued that through laying responsibility on the suffering, much of the conflictual political energy caused by structural inequality was consciously being undermined by those whose interests are served by the status quo. Although biomedical science recognizes that health and illness result from the interaction of numerous causative factors, this multi-factorial perspective was jettisoned in planning preventive strategies through the 1970s and 1980s, restricting health promoters to a narrow behavioural focus (Jackson 1985).

The critique of victim-blaming in health promotion draws on the work of William Ryan, who showed that this process happens in all areas of social conflict and its formula for operation appears quite smooth:

> First, identify a social problem. Second, study those affected by the problem and discover in what ways they are different from the rest of us as a consequence of deprivation and injustice. Third, define the differences as the cause of the social problem itself. Finally, [...] assign a government bureaucrat to invent a humanitarian action program to correct the differences.
>
> (Ryan 1976: 8–9)

Ryan explored the ways in which a range of social services, from psychiatry to schooling, identify personality of cultural traits in disempowered groups and hold these responsible for the poor social situation of the group. He assumes that all such cultural factors are the effects of structural powerlessness, without giving any alternative theorization of the relationship between the objective causes (poverty, racism, social exclusion) and the subjective effects (less interest in education, lower self-esteem, higher rates of mental illnesses). Crawford recognized in the 1970s that the American health-care system was beginning to understand the social production of ill health and at the same time realizing that the medical system was a costly and ineffective means of improving the health of a population. The individual responsibility arguments which were proposed as a way out of this crisis, Crawford observed, tend to ignore the social and environmental causes of illness and employ an 'unrealistic' model of human behaviour.

The promises of the 1970s that self-care would provide a way of reining in escalating health-care costs now appear rather simplistic. It is perhaps impossible to determine the overall economic impacts of the interest in self-care, given the cost-shifting involved and the inherent complexities of measuring the economic impacts of health-care interventions. For example, spending money on a media campaign to educate the public about the symptoms of mental illnesses may result in an increased demand for psychiatric services. There may be broader economic benefits involved but these are extremely difficult to calculate (Mooney 1995). Many institutional purchasers of health care – governments and health insurance companies – are obviously convinced that in certain circumstances it is cost-effective for them to spend vast amounts of money on self-care promotion campaigns. This is especially the case in smoking cessation campaigns by governments and accident prevention campaigns by insurance companies.

What is clear is that consumer spending on self-care has increased considerably. There has been a huge growth since the 1970s in sales of self-help books, gym memberships, sporting equipment, vitamin supplements, and so on. In many cases health-care providers have indeed been able to shift the burden of care onto consumers, resulting in substantial cost reductions. This is readily apparent, for example, in early discharge policies, which have shortened hospital stays for a wide range of procedures, thus reducing costs for hospitals while increasing the demands made on patients' families. The amount spent on health as a whole, though, has shown no sign of diminishing.

7 Narcissism and self-care

Theorizing America's obsession with mundane health behaviour

Dark as the grave, that's how my heart is
Like water flowing from a spring, that's how my tears flow
When you've burnt out, heart of mine, I'll gather up the ashes
And I'll make a potion for healing hearts
Stratis Galathianakis, 'Daybreak Syrtos' (Apodimi Compania 1992)

A new popular health consciousness seemed to emerge in the United States during the late 1960s and 1970s. There was a surge in interest in personal health and well-being, expressed in a wide variety of health-related social movements (including vegetarianism, the natural health movement, the women's health movement and consumerist critiques of medical practice) and consumer fads (grapefruit juice, aerobics, workout videos, etc.). It seemed as though the mundane world of self-care had become a national obsession. The myriad day-to-day practices that individuals engage in to recover, maintain or improve their health had become topics worthy of public discourse, filling the shelves of book-shops and newsagents and becoming a constant preoccupation on talk-back radio and in the lifestyle programming that flooded television schedules.

Today, personal striving and spending to improve health are taken for granted. In the 1970s, however, when self-care practices were new to the public sphere and the market, there was much discussion of the meaning of these new obsessions. People were divided over the appropriateness of discussing intimate details in public, such as the colour of one's urine, the contents of one's refrigerator or the frequency of one's orgasms. To some, such pettiness reeked of self-obsession, leading Tom Wolfe to famously call the 1970s 'the me decade' (cited in Lasch 1980: 5). For others, the body had been liberated from decades of repression. In order better to understand the society we live in today, it is worth revisiting these debates, which were carried out at a time when the public cele-bration of the mundane was still shocking and exciting. It is difficult to be shocked or excited any longer. This era is not only of interest for Americans. With the exportation of American popular culture, these petty conundrums have been globalized. These developments in 1970s America had repercussions across the world, especially in English-speaking societies, where the influence of American popular culture is greatest. Around the world there have been similar intellectual debates, in which writers have tried to understand the meaning of such public mundanities. These debates have paralleled those within the United States. The only difference is that while Americans see such phenomena as peculiarly Californian, the rest of the world sees such a focus on the self as peculiarly American.

As was discussed in Chapter 5, on the Left, popular interest in self-care was interpreted as part of an anti-institutional critique of medicine. Writers such as Ivan Illich (1976) and Irving Zola (1972, 1973) saw self-care as a force against professional dependency. Their critique of institutionalized health care closely followed Parsons' functionalist understanding of the medical profession. They saw professional-institutional forms of health care as mechanisms of social control and so saw the rise of self-care as the expression of a popular liberatory rebellion against institutional power. This interpretation fitted neatly with the early consumer backlash against medicine and psychiatry in the 1960s and 1970s. One broad theme in many of these movements was an effort to reduce dependency on professional health-care services and institutions by providing individuals with tools to undertake their own self-care.

The other major intellectual response to the appearance of these self-active cultural forms was the critique of cultural narcissism, which I will discuss in this chapter. Best known through the work of Philip Rieff (1966), Richard Sennett (1974) and Christopher Lasch (1980, 1984), this tradition of disparaging and often despairing intellectual comment on what are seen as the self-obsessional tendencies promoted by consumer capitalism has been a major influence on subsequent critical interpretations of popular interest in mundane health behaviour. While the anti-institutional writers tended to confine their discussion to the relationships between individuals and health-care institutions, the critics of narcissism were more broadly concerned with the rise of diverse forms of intro-spectivity in popular culture. They were critical of what they saw as a new type of inward-looking personality. Instead of celebrating self-care as resistance to medical dominance, as Illich and Zola had done, these writers saw the rise of self-care practices in popular culture as evidence of a variety of forms of social decay.

Critiques of cultural narcissism often focused on extraordinary new counter-cultural movements that appeared to be particularly self-obsessed. Peter Marin (1975), writing in *Harper's* magazine, described the self-religions that were later to call themselves the New Age movement (see also Heelas 1996). He recounts a conversation he had with a man who had embraced mysticism and spirituality.

> He was telling me about his sense of another reality.
> 'I know there is something outside of me,' he said. 'I can feel it. I know it is there. But what is it?'
> 'It may not be a mystery,' I said. 'Perhaps it is the world.'
>
> (Marin 1975: 50)

Marin argues that the worlds of community, history and social action have been so eroded that people have only the inner world in which to find meaning, and social life appears to them as a mystical recollection of a world beyond the self.

At the same time as these fringe cultures were causing concern to some intellectuals, the mass media became focused on the private self in ways that were perhaps less spiritual, but were seen as equally narcissistic. Why, the critics asked, have Americans become so preoccupied with such mundane aspects of their private lives?

Diagnosing social forms

Lasch, Rieff and Sennett argue that structural changes in American society were changing individuals' psychology, leading to a shift in the dominant personality type of the society as a whole. The tradition of psychoanalytic diagnosis of culture dates at least from Freud, but theories of fundamental contradictions between human nature and society are of course much older. Marx's 'species nature', for example, was based on his notion of the spontaneously arisen natural community, and in part his theories of alienation in class society centre on the incompatibility between this species nature and the psychic requirements of the capitalist mode of production. Freud (1985) later theorized a fundamental contradiction between human nature (the id or the pleasure principle) and culture (the ego or reality principle). The 'polymorphous perversity' of primary human nature, he argued, is incompatible with the cooperative requirements of civilized societies:

> We cannot fail to be struck by the similarity between the process of civilization and the libidinal development of the individual. [...] Sublimation of instinct is an especially conspicuous feature of cultural development; it is what makes it possible for higher psychical activities, scientific, artistic, or ideological, to play such an important part in civilized life.
>
> (Freud 1985: 286)

Freud could see no way out of this fundamental conflict, since the more civilized a society becomes, the greater the repression required. The non-satisfaction of powerful instincts results in hostility in every society, and in neurosis.

In Germany in the 1930s, the welding of psychoanalysis with Marxism led to a number of psycho-sociological explorations of the modern psyche. Even before Adorno and Reich had attempted to explain the rise of fascism in psychoanalytic terms, Karen Horney (1937) had written one of the first overtly psychological diagnoses of modernity. In *The Neurotic Personality of Our Time* she sees the root of neuroses in the fears and conflicting tendencies inherent in her culture. She lists as the most important of these cultural conflicts those between competition and brotherly love; between desires and their dissatisfaction; and between alleged freedom and actual limitations (Horney 1937: 288–9). Most people, she observed, manage to negotiate these contradictions and accept them as part of 'modern living', while those who cannot are diagnosed as neurotic. These three tensions arise from the relatively free-floating nature of modern life as compared with the more predetermined and restrictive conditions of more traditional social forms. These tensions have been intensified since Horney wrote, and they form the central themes of this thesis, to the extent that self-care promotion is involved in shaping individuals' personal negotiations of the tensions between selfishness and cooperation; desires and dissatisfaction; and perceived freedom and actual limitations.

Decades later in the United States, the psychological conflict between the individual and the civilized society once more came to the fore. During the 1950s and 1960s many American social commentators wrote of the perceived loss of individual autonomy in the face of the homogenizing and depersonalizing effects of 'mass society', in many ways echoing Weber's writings on rationalization. These critiques responded to the increasing influence of professional-institutional modes of practice, in which the power held by the mass media, big business, big government and big unions was seen to threaten those individualistic values – self-reliance, independence and personal initiative – which were held up as the motive force of the American dream. With the heavy influence of psychology, and especially psychoanalysis, on American social criticism in this period, the emerging 'mass society' was seen to be moulding a new type of psychological make-up. David Riesman, for example, identified two ideal-typical personality structures, the inner-directed and the other-directed. The inner-directed person is typified by the self-reliant individual of the nineteenth century. This personality type internalizes cultural imperatives, using them as a resource in acting independently. Riesman argued that the inner-directed personality had given way to the other-directed, heteronomous personality type, and he feared the gradual loss of individuality in the face of the conformism that was resulting (Riesman *et al.* 1950). He asserted that individual defences are battered down by 'the group', despite the persistence of a contradictory and increasingly anachronistic ideology of free-enterprise and individualism. The critiques of medicalization offered by Illich and Zola were heavily influenced by the broader analysis of the loss of personal autonomy in the face of professional-institutional modes of practice.

The emergence of the 'counter-culture' in the late 1960s in the United States, with its heavy emphasis on introspective self-exploration, was in part an oppositional reaction to the 'mass society'. The 1950s precursors to the counter-culture, the Beats, thought of themselves as spiritual refugees fleeing the uniformity and boredom of suburbia, or, as Kerouac explained, from 'the people watching television, the millions and millions of the One Eye' (Kerouac 1958: 104). Instead the Beats sought mobility and extremes, wild experiences to escape from the predictability of suburban life. They were on a search for meaning and spirit in what they saw as a heartless world, and for a way of living more meaningfully. They were drawn together by their desire to elude the mainstream and to avoid angst by resorting to hyper-mobility. They looked to Zen Buddhism to provide deeper inspiration and meaning to their escapism and to guide the perpetual search for new experiences (see Ziguras 1997a). Vytautas Kavolas (1970), writing about the psychological make-up of 'post-modern man', expresses most clearly the approach which sees the dominant 'modern' and oppositional 'underground' personality types as both derived from social structural changes – the one reflecting what Parsons might have termed systemic imperatives and the other a reaction to these forces:

> If the sociological trend [...] is toward an increasingly rationalized and impersonal bureaucracy, its psychological resultant may be a more rationally organized and unemotionally performing type of personality, concerned only with the orderly application of rules rather than with the solution of immediate existential or ultimate philosophical problems. But, *as a reaction to* the sociological trend, an exaggeratedly irrational kind of personality might emerge – one inclined toward anarchic romanticism, expressionism, mysticism, and the politics and education of 'ecstasy'.
>
> (Kavolas 1970: 436)

The desire of many young people to 'drop out' of mainstream society in the late 1960s and early 1970s in the United States, much noted by mainstream writers at the time, was only one side of the process. The critics of narcissism tended to overlook the other side of this process, which was captured in the 'tune in, turn on' part of Timothy Leary's famous exhortation. T.R. Young, to pick one of thousands of possible examples, told his readers in 1970 that 'modern society has become much too flimsy a fabric out of which to build a self-system', encouraging readers to turn instead to 'new sources of self'. These include 'the next generation of psychiatrists, clinical psychologists, and psychiatric social workers [who] will "help" us to be unattached rather than adjusted to the social order' (Young 1972: x, 1). He encouraged the rejection of 'society' in favour of self-constitution, with the aid of those new sources.

An inward turn?

While young people were turning to these 'new sources of self', social commentators tended to focus on the loss of the old sources of self. In 1957, a team of American social researchers conducted what amounted to a psychological profile of the American population, which was then repeated in 1976. Between 1957 and 1976 they observed 'a *reduced integration of American adults into the social structure*', and saw this as 'a shift from a *socially* integrated paradigm for structuring well-being, to a more *personal* or individual paradigm' (cited in Collier 1991: 224). This shift was accompanied by a higher degree of introspection and a tendency to visit others less and belong to fewer organizations. A similar study, led by Robert Bellah, particularly interested in the relationship between private and public life, suggested that an 'expressive' or 'lifestyle' individualism had replaced the earlier utilitarian or economic individualism. The new individualism was putting in jeopardy the survival of democratic institutions, which, the researchers argued, depend on

> the extent to which private life either prepares people to take part in the public world or encourages them to find meaning exclusively in the private sphere, and the degree to which public life fulfils our private aspirations or discourages us so much that we withdraw from involvement in it.
>
> (Bellah *et al.* 1985: ix)

They argued that work continued to be centrally important to the self-identity of Americans and their concern with self-reliance, so the work ethic remained strong, but was now accompanied by an isolating preoccupation with the self (Bellah *et al.* 1985: 56). Rieff, Sennett and Lasch drew upon such empirical studies to argue that a narcissistic form of individualism that celebrates self-expression and self-gratification was replacing the rugged individualism of the nineteenth century (Lasch 1980: xv). While those involved in the new social and cultural movements saw opportunities for growth, exploration and transformation in the new tools for rethinking the mundane, conservative critics such as Lasch saw the growing interest in practices of the self as an inward turn that involved the withdrawal from the social or public sphere and a narcissistic and solipsistic obsession with the inner self.

Sennett wrote in *The Fall of Public Man* that impersonal relations in the public sphere were increasingly seen as phoney obligations, causing people to turn to their private lives for authenticity and meaning. Intimacy and private life were coming to be seen as ends in themselves, and the psyche was 'treated as if it had a life of its own' (Sennett 1974: 4). Sennett believed that one result of the preoccupation with the self was confusion between public and intimate life. Increasingly, people were dealing with public matters in terms of personal feelings – matters that he believed could only properly be dealt with through codes of impersonal meaning. This confusion of boundaries between the self and the external world, between the private and public spheres, was a major concern for the critics of narcissism, for a number of reasons:

1   Democracy was seen to rest on the ability of citizens to rise above self-interest in order to act for the public good, and this blurring raised the fear that people would no longer be able to think beyond their own self-interest.
2   The public seemed to be more interested in their leaders' private lives than their political actions.
3   These critics did not welcome the politicization of the private sphere. Being well-educated white middle-class men, they were members of the most privileged segment of the population – those with most to lose from the politicization of the interpersonal relations with regard to gender, race or class.

It is now fashionable to deconstruct the public–private dichotomy as a fiction complicit in the maintenance of established power relations. Nikolas Rose, for example, states: 'The distinction between public and private is not a stable analytical tool, but is itself a mobile resource in these systems of knowledge and power' (Rose 1990: 217). While this may be true, it begs the question of why this 'fiction' held up for so long, and has only become visible as an imaginary construct relatively recently. The distinction between public and private did indeed serve as a *stable* analytical tool until very recently. It has become a *mobile* resource primarily because the relative autonomy of these spheres has been seriously eroded. The value of Lasch, Rieff and Sennett's work is in theorizing this shifting of boundaries so that the mundane details of private life suddenly became worthy of public exposure.

The mediation of the mundane

These commentators were witnessing the birth of new therapies, new forms of expertise, new types of radio programmes and new dietary fads. People have always been involved in the types of self-care that were the focus of these 'new sources of self', but previously these mundane conversations had been conducted in the privacy of one's house or one's own head. Now they were being broadcast, bought and sold, and studied as never before. These writers see the media's interest in the private self as a major influence in eroding public life in America. Sennett, for example, lays some of the blame at the feet of electronic media:

> Electronic communication is one means by which the very idea of public life has been put to an end. The media have vastly increased the store of knowledge social groups have about each other, but have rendered actual contact unnecessary. The radio, and more especially the TV, are intimate devices; mostly you watch them at home.
>
> (Sennett, 1974: 282)

These commentators the media and professional interest in mundane self-care as separating people from one another, facilitating a withdrawal from social interaction. This sentiment is expressed powerfully by James Lincoln Collier, who claims that the increasing amount of time Americans spend in front of television is a major cause of what he calls the rise of selfishness in America:

> What is troubling about this enormous immersion in television and the media in general, is the extent to which it has isolated people one from one another. At bottom, television is a machine which helps people to wall themselves off from one another. So long as we are engaged with the magic box, we are not engaged with others.
>
> (Collier 1991: 245)

What Collier forgets is that while TV watchers may not be engaged in face-to-face interaction with others, they are certainly involved in a form of communication with others. Lasch, Rieff and Sennett also focus on the erosion of face-to-face interaction and generally miss the fact that self-care practices are increasingly reconstituted through mediated communications with others.

While these writers focused on the mental health implications for individuals, they generally overlooked the production and dissemination of mediated self-care advice. One early exception was Arthur Brittan, who in *The Privatised World* described the 'invasion of consciousness' as a process of privatization in which 'the subjective experience of individuals in industrialised and capitalist societies is distorted and influenced by the mass media and bureaucracy' (Brittan 1977: 147). He emphasizes the extent to which the private sphere is reconstituted by mediated information, so that even the most intimate aspects of private life have become the subject of public discussion:

> Sexual privacy, supposedly an essential requirement of personal identity, is now subject to the dispassionate analysis of experts who comment on technique, performance and impotence, to a world-wide audience who suddenly discover their own sexual inadequacies. [...] Sexual privacy is, therefore, an illusion because each sexual episode is geared into a vast network of performance requirements, which in turn generate anxiety about the sexual adequacy of the participants.
>
> (Brittan 1977: 147)

Brittan argues that the analysis of this situation is torn between mental health analyses that see this emphasis on the private lives of individuals as narcissism, as the writers I am considering do, or else as media manipulation, as Frankfurt School social theorists such as Horkheimer (1972) and Althusser (1969) had done. Both of these approaches tended to see the individual as being in a vulnerable and unhappy situation, as did the Foucauldian approaches to this issue in the late 1980s and 1990s (see, for example, Rose 1990; Lupton 1995).

The loss of religious authority over the mundane

The critics of narcissism saw the popular demand for self-care advice as being fuelled by a deep void – a loss of meaning generally attributed to a loss of religious faith, a distrust for authority, and the fragmentation of close-knit social relations in favour of looser connections. Philip Rieff argued in *The Triumph of the Therapeutic* (1966) that the power of psychologically trained professionals was causing a shift in the dominant culture of Western societies, from a 'Christian culture' to a 'therapeutic culture'. The emergence of psychological man was one of the effects of the collapse of 'Christian culture' and its attendant institutions, which, he argued, had previously saved believers from 'destructive illusions of uniqueness and separateness' (Rieff 1966: 3). Rieff proposed that whereas

[r]eligious man was born to be saved, psychological man is born to be pleased. The difference was established long ago, when 'I believe', the cry of the ascetic, lost preference to 'one feels', the caveat of the therapeutic. And if the therapeutic is to win out, then surely the psychotherapist will be his secular spiritual guide.

(Rieff 1966: 24–5)

Rieff may be exaggerating the hold which psychoanalysis and humanistic psychology had over the fields of psychology and psychiatry as a whole in this period, when behaviourism was becoming dominant in mainstream psychology. Nevertheless, he points to a dramatic shift in professional practice to align professional expertise with the self-care capacities of the patient, so that rather than surrendering to the professional and 'following doctor's orders', the practitioner and patient began to work together and alongside one another in a cooperative manner.

Paul Halmos (1970) developed Rieff's thesis in more detail, arguing that the 'personal service professions', as he terms them, have developed a relatively coherent counselling ideology. He groups professionals into either 'personal service professions' (clergy, doctors, nurses, teachers, social workers) or 'impersonal service professions' (lawyers, accountants, engineers, architects). The principal function of personal service professions, he states, is to 'bring about changes in the body or personality of the client' by implementing techniques applied from the social and psychological sciences (Halmos 1970: 22). Whereas Rieff saw all professional intervention in psychological and emotional realms which was not of a religious orientation as therapeutic, even describing political ideologies such as Marxism as 'therapies of commitment', Halmos distinguishes between 'reformist' and 'therapeutic' interventions, where reformist orientations attempt 'to change the rules which regulate social relationships' and therapeutic orientations aim to 'change the personality of the client or the patient' (Halmos 1970: 18). Halmos argued that the therapeutic approaches to dealing with personal problems were not merely a result of the professionalization of self-care advice, but must also be studied in terms of the nature of the dominant ideologies within such professions.

Before the advent of new forms of expertise on the mundane aspects of daily life (pop-psychology, health and fitness experts, alternative therapies), the only public institutions to deal in any depth with such matters were religious authorities. Now the clerics had lost ground in the battle to shape dietary, emotional and sexual practices.

Lasch also argued that the religious desire for salvation by surrendering oneself to a higher power had given way to the desire for well-being and health, which is to be achieved through the taking of control over one's self rather than surrendering it. In contrast to Rieff, however, Lasch contended that therapy constituted an anti-religion. While religions construct a moral realm that extends far beyond the space and time occupied by the person, modern societies cannot envisage anything beyond immediate needs, and therapeutic cultures can conceive of nothing beyond the immediate desires of the individual (Lasch 1980: 7–13). On one side of the division of labour between religion and psychology, therapy substituted religious salvation with the attainment of a desirable mental state, variously referring to this state as self-actualization, happiness or wholeness. Meanwhile, on the religious side of this divide, new religious movements with decidedly therapeutic approaches emerged. The New Age movement is a loose collection of such 'self-religions' that treat the inner self as the ultimate source of contentment and well-being. The self is conceived as a quasi-spiritual entity, existing on a different plane and requiring transcendent practices in order to be reached (Heelas 1982, 1996).

Lasch argues that because of the loss of stable sources of authority, those in narcissistic societies are increasingly dependent on celebrities, media personalities, professionals, experts and bureaucracies for validation. The lack of deep engagement with others leads to the individual's craving for approval and admiration, and this need cannot be satisfied by the fleeting or absent others from whom it is sought.

> His [*sic*] apparent freedom from family ties and institutional constraints does not free him to stand alone or to glory in his individuality. On the contrary, it contributes to his insecurity, which he can overcome only by seeing his 'grandiose self' reflected in the attentions of others, or by attaching himself to those who radiate celebrity, power and charisma.
>
> (Lasch 1980: 10)

In contrast to the reliance on one's family, this is a 'new paternalism', a dependence encouraged by professionals and bureaucracies. In turn, these institutional agents transform collective grievances into personal issues amenable to therapeutic intervention (Lasch 1980: 14). In his later work, Lasch (1984) increasingly casts reflexive practices of the self as mere coping mechanisms. He argues that people have turned inward because of the desperate state of a world threatened by environmental disasters, nuclear apocalypse, decaying cities and other seemingly intractable crises over which the person has no control. Crisis, he argues, has been normalized to the extent that people no longer expect to be able to make sense of the world or to find a meaningful existence with reference to once reliable meta-narratives or institutions. Narcissism is thus a defensive strategy, a reaction against fears of abandonment and feelings of anxiety and guilt.

The loss of social support

As well as mourning the loss of more authoritative forms of religious practice, the critics of narcissism mourn the loss of face-to-face community and the sense of meaning and belonging afforded by such a community. In the earlier culture, which is being displaced by the therapeutic culture, there were positive psychological, religious and ethical rewards for pro-social behaviour, good citizenship and communal values that were mutually reinforcing. In this culture, according to Rieff, there was 'a design of motives directing the self outward, toward those communal purposes in which alone the self can be realized and satisfied' (Rieff 1966: 4). In modern industrial societies however, the bonds between each person in the chain of social responsibility are being broken, so that everybody lives a truly private life, and individualistic philosophies that attempt to make sense of this condition increasingly take hold. Therapeutic systems are seen as a response to a loss of faith.

The emergent therapeutic culture attempts to soothe the descent into meaninglessness experienced by late modern subjects. Rieff, Sennett and Lasch, however, contend that the therapeutic remedies actually exacerbate the social problems they seek to cure. They argue that the forms of community that exist in individualistic societies are not strong enough to establish a positive culture. Rieff concludes that the desire for freedom is self-defeating. Satisfaction, he argues (perhaps rather anachronistically), can only be attained by surrender to a higher power, an unquestioned designer of communal purposes. This religious critique of self-care is often encountered in conservative responses to contemporary cultural issues of many kinds.

Lasch likewise interprets the narcissist's obsession with the self as a desperate search for the means to counter the insecurity produced by the weakening of the social super-ego that was formerly represented by the father, teachers and preachers. The rugged individual of the nineteenth century could act confidently in the world because these sources of authority could be taken for granted. In contrast, Lasch argues, the 'psychological man' of the twentieth century searches desperately for a personal peace of mind while the social and personal conditions of contemporary life make that end increasingly hard to achieve (see also Rose 1990: 216). Lasch sees the preoccupation with consciousness as an indication that there is a void within which creates a desire for therapeutic interventions. Rather than a hedonistic pursuit of pleasure for its own sake, he sees contemporary demands for therapeutic assistance as part of a 'struggle for composure' by individuals who feel lost or fragmented. However, this recourse to expert help is thoroughly self-defeating, according to Lasch. Therapeutic approaches that seek to counter this sense of meaninglessness by helping the person to overcome their inhibitions and helping them in satisfying their desires only heighten the individualization of the person, exacerbating the problems of disconnection they experience. Lasch characterizes all therapeutic systems as advocating social withdrawal, and so sees 'the consciousness movement' as inherently self-defeating:

> Arising out of a pervasive dissatisfaction with the quality of personal relations, it advises people not to make too large an investment in love and friendship, to avoid excessive dependence on others, and to live for the moment – the very conditions that created the crisis of personal relations in the first place.
>
> (Lasch 1980: 27)

To use the example of love, according to Lasch, in the therapeutic enterprise love is discussed in terms of the emotional self-interest of the patient rather than to encourage the individual to subordinate their needs to those of others. Because of the self-interested nature of such a relationship, the resulting emotional attachment lacks meaning, according to Lasch, when compared with more traditional notions of love as self-sacrifice and self-abasement. The meaningfulness of relationships in earlier times was conveyed by the requirement for self-sacrifice for the other, or submission to a higher loyalty (Lasch 1980: 13). Lasch here characterizes all therapeutic advice as encouraging a withdrawal from interpersonal relationships. He ignores those types of therapy that work to help the person reintegrate themselves with a network of caring others and to rebuild damaged relationships.

Arlie Russel Hochschild (1994) analysed the degree to which contemporary women's self-help literature encourages its readers to withdraw from social relationships (which she calls 'cool' advice) or to engage more fully with others ('warm' advice) in order to overcome various life crises. Warm and cool forms of advice differ in their attitudes to emotional investment. Warm advice emphasizes the desirability of connectedness, stability and safety, whereas cool advice values positively individual freedom, self-sufficiency and disengagement. Hochschild sees a distinct contrast between the generally warm tendencies of the self-help books advocating 'traditional' gender identities and the cool tendencies of those favouring feminist-informed 'modern' identities. Many of the 'cool moderns', as Hochschild terms them, argue that the desire to be safe and warm is the cause of women's problems. Conspicuous as one of the few warm moderns is the early feminist self-care book, *Our Bodies Ourselves*, published by the Boston Women's Health Book Collective in 1971. It retains the communitarian emphasis of the political wing of the counter-culture that is not so evident in later self-help publishing. This feature of much self-help literature is at the centre of a number of debates on the political significance of such individualizing self-care discourses, and will form the basis of much of the discussion in later chapters.

While her overall conclusions reinforce Lasch's argument, Hochschild does remind us that advice (whether delivered by a professional or a text) is able to encourage social integration just as it can advocate withdrawal. Lasch often characterizes therapy as inevitably anti-social, but at other times concedes that such 'warm' and sociologically informed forms of advice-giving are possible. A productive form of therapy, he argues, would involve providing critical insights into a person's condition so they can 'gain insight into the historical forces, reproduced in psychological form, that have made the concept of selfhood increasingly problematic' (Lasch 1980: 17). Giddens likewise observes that therapy is not simply 'a means of adjusting dissatisfied individuals to a flawed social environment' but instead is often a proactive method of life-planning which responds in appropriate ways to the 'dislocations and uncertainties to which modernity gives rise' (Giddens 1991: 180).

Lasch and the other critics of narcissism tend to focus too heavily on the consumption of self-care and overlook its production. They read contemporary culture by looking at the assumed audience written into texts by the producers of such self-help cultures. In this they perhaps overstate the fears and cravings of American society. (They are like the Martians who study life on earth by intercepting television transmissions.) I think it is necessary to also look at the conditions of production of self-care in order to understand the phenomenon. If, on the demand side of self-care promotion, audiences are retreating into themselves, on the supply side, the production of culture is penetrating deeper into the person also. The critics of narcissism see the contemporary self illuminated in the more visible cultural forms. Intimate discussions over a coffee table are not as visible to the cultural critic as intimate articles in magazines, and with the integration of the self now occurring on more abstract levels, the culture appears to be self-obsessed. The culture may in fact be no more self-obsessed than it has ever been, but the way its self-obsession is worked out through professional and mediated relationships is much more striking to the cultural critic. Since the 1970s, social life has changed in ways that make the distinction between public and private acts impossible to sustain analytically. The separation between a private sphere framed by face-to-face interaction and a public sphere composed of institutions and abstract relationships has been eroded. The media and new forms of expertise ignore the separation of public and private, detraditionalizing the mundane care of the self and turning it into a battleground to be fought over by numerous interest groups. What this discussion has shown us, I believe, is the value of empirical studies of consumers of mediated health information. People often gather information and advice strategically, deciding which sources to consult and how to weigh the information they obtain from various sources. They may consult friends, health-care professionals, advertising material, self-help books, magazines and, now, the Internet (A. Rogers *et al.* 1999). The media do not mirror the nation's soul, and theorists who attempt to describe social practices based on an analysis of mediated content often underestimate the agency of the audience.

To some social critics, the preponderance of self-help texts represented a growing introversion and the emergence of a self-obsessed culture. This was hardly a 'withdrawal' into the self, however. Rather, the reflexive concerns of the private person were made very public in the mass media. And as the private issues of the self exploded into public life, numerous political and therapeutic self-care philosophies responded to the anxieties caused by the detraditionalization of lifestyle.

8 Governing one's self

[W]hat authority is claimed by those who have acquired the power to speak the truth about persons, to provide truthful answers to the question of how one should live, how one should direct or remake one's life?

Nikolas Rose, 'Authority and the genealogy of subjectivity' (1996: 301)

Michel Foucault's work has been extremely influential in shaping sociological understandings of self-care. Most significant of the 1990s Foucauldians was Nikolas Rose, who theorized the ways in which 'governance', in its broadest sense, increasingly shapes the self-active capacities of autonomous individuals in order to instil desired behaviours. This chapter examines the contribution of poststructuralist critiques of neo-liberal self-care promotion. A number of writers who have adopted a 'governmentality' approach have discussed the relationship between activating technologies and what they refer to as the neo-liberal mode of government, which involves the reorientation of state activity away from the provision of security to the activation of an entrepreneurial and striving citizen.

In Foucault's writings there are two different forms of the application of expertise to the self, which are made most explicit in his dual use of the term 'government'. Government refers broadly to 'the conduct of conduct', but more specifically to the calculated and methodical ways of shaping behaviour. These are characteristically modern behavioural technologies drawing on institutional expertise to govern behaviour instrumentally. On the one hand, Foucault refers to the ways in which institutions use expert systems to govern the behaviour of their subjects – the technologization of the management of others. On the other hand, the reflexive management of the self has been technologized as a consequence of the application of techniques developed by expert systems. Foucault to these as 'techniques of domination' and 'techniques of the self', respectively.

Much of Foucault's earlier work is concerned with the former of these – the less reflexive 'modes of objectification which transform human beings into subjects' (Foucault 1982: 777). This dimension of governmentality, in Rose and Miller's elaboration of the concept, refers to 'the historically constituted matrix within which are articulated all those dreams, schemes, strategies and manoeuvres of authorities that seek to shape the beliefs and conduct of others in desired directions by acting upon their will, their circumstances or their environment' (Rose and Miller 1992: 175). The technologies of *domination* that Foucault describes in *Discipline and Punish* (1977) were used to extract utility from a body that was rendered docile. Foucault's later work on the history of sexuality shifts its emphasis to the reflexive dimension of governmentality – the 'way a human being turns himself [*sic*] into a subject' (Foucault 1982: 778). These technologies of the *self* are means of consciously working upon one's self which 'permit individuals to effect by their own means or with the help of others a certain number of operations on their bodies and souls, thoughts, conduct, and a way of being, so as to transform themselves' (Foucault 1988: 18). The reflexive technologies of the self allow one to acquire mastery over one's own body, but this is possible 'only through the effect of an investment of power in the body' (Foucault 1980: 56). These dual interests are difficult to reconcile as they are given different emphasis in different texts. *Discipline and Punish* presents an overly structuralist treatment of objectification, focusing on the production of docile bodies, while in Foucault's later works on the history of sexuality there is a dramatic shift in emphasis to the project of reflexive self-formation through technologies of the self. Partly because of this development of his ideas, the relationship between these two processes is never clearly developed.

In Foucault's work on the rise of disciplinary power, he charted the growing influence of what I am calling the professional-institutional level of social integration. Previously, 'sovereign power' had operated mainly through restriction – by delimiting permitted and forbidden behaviour. While transgression may have been harshly punished, sovereign power was little interested in the conduct of the everyday lives of subjects, as long as they did not flout the law. Disciplinary power, however, represented a new logic of control. Whereas sovereign power was restrictive, disciplinary power is productive, attempting to shape behaviour through the use of a vast array of techniques that make possible the organized and instrumental reformulation of spheres of life previously of little interest to powerful institutions.

There had long been arts of the human body directed at the 'growth of skills', but what was new about disciplinary coercion, according to Foucault, was that it established 'in the body the constricting link between an increased aptitude and an increased domination' (Foucault 1977: 137–8). He was later to refer to this more continuous and corrective management of the conduct of life as biopower, a term which emphasizes his view that the body was a primary object of disciplinary regimes (Foucault 1981). Rather than seeing the body as a physiological constant, he put forward a social constructionism, seeing the body as affected by 'history' in the sense that it is 'broken down by a great many distinct regimes' (cited in Crossley 1996: 101). Biopower operated through disciplinary techniques directed at both an individual and a population level. At the individual level, Foucault describes an 'anatomo-politics of the human body' which 'centred on the body as machine: its disciplining, the optimization of its capabilities, the exertion of its forces, the parallel increase of its usefulness and its docility, its integration into systems of efficient and economic controls'. On the population level, biopower operated through regulatory controls 'serving as the basis of the biological processes: propagation, births and mortalities, the level of health, life expectancy and longevity, with all the conditions which caused these to vary' (Foucault 1981: 139). Foucault sought to demonstrate how these regimes that developed in the factory, the prison, the army and the hospital had been applied far beyond the walls of these institutions and had come to permeate the social whole.

Foucault is almost silent on the question of 'social control' before the advent of disciplinary power over self-care. In failing to account for pre-disciplinary forms of social integration, it appears in his work as if the 'private' dimensions of the person are not touched by power until such modern institutions develop. This leads to a tendency to treat the subject as a blank slate before the exercise of disciplinary powers. In equating power with the state's means of ruling populations, Foucault glosses over the fact that cultural codes, transmitted at the face-to-face level, also play a part in the constitution of subjectivity. What he observes is the development of more institutionalized techniques for ordering social life that were incorporated into the modern state's regulation of bodies in a systematized manner. These disciplinary techniques overlay and often contradict with the more culturally embedded modes of constitution of self-care practices.

Foucault touches on some of these issues in his work on the history of sexuality, mainly in his discussions of the role of the confessional in the Catholic Church and the operation of classical self-help texts. Organized religions were some of the earliest manifestations of professional-institutional integration, in which the clergy acted as relatively impersonal representatives or agents for an abstract system with its own rules and expertise. They relied on the authority of holy texts that drew on the religiosity of a certain culture and froze it in time, so that the monotheistic religions today still reflect to some extent the cultural – including dietary and self-care – practices of the writers of those texts. As these institutions expanded their reach, they absorbed certain local practices and abolished others. While Foucault's analysis of the confessional is interesting as a study of an early form of this type of abstract relationship between authority figure and lay public, here, too, he tends to ignore the face-to-face culture in which the clergy operated (Foucault 1981). The later volumes of the history of sexuality series involve a close reading of a number of texts which offer instructions for the conduct of everyday life to the ancient Greek and Roman elites (Foucault 1990a, 1990b). Similar self-help texts were of course produced in Asia, but what all of these had in common was a relatively small readership due to the difficulty of producing manuscripts and the low levels of literacy. For my purposes here, the most interesting thing about these texts is the relationship between the expert knowledge that was written in them and the popular knowledge which was never written down, but which played a far more important role in shaping the self-care practices of the mass of the population. My point is that the neither the sovereign, the clergy, nor the philosophers were the major forces shaping the conduct of everyday life before the advent of modern disciplinary apparatuses.

If the body is a product of history, as Foucault states, then it is necessary to explain how embodiment was constituted prior to the development of disciplinary techniques. His later work on the history of sexuality does analyse the self-help literatures of the literate elites in antiquity, but these reached very small audiences, and, because of their literary and therefore more consciously reflexive form, were already a different type of integration when compared with the face-to-face constitution of embodiment.

Foucault's observations are more useful when seen in the context of broad processes of detraditionalization, in which modernization dissolves traditional ways of life, overlaying them with behaviours shaped by expert systems. Traditional self-care practices are deeply integrated into local cultures, forming part of a community's collective memory. These traditional self-care practices come to be undermined by modern practices whose genesis is very different. The regimes that Foucault is interested in are technologized in the sense that they involve the application of an organized body of knowledge to specific tasks. Because of the universalizing aspirations of modern expert systems and their more organized and calculating institutional transmission, modern self-care techniques override the localism of face-to-face forms. Simultaneously, more and more spheres of life are addressed by expert systems that produce technologies for reconfiguring these behaviours. We can say, then, that disciplinary power represents the rise to prominence of a more abstract level of social integration, which overlays but does not replace the face-to-face level of integration.

Foucault used the model of the panopticon to emphasize the way in which discursive power operates through internalizing behavioural norms in subjects who are aware of being scrutinized. The normalized self maintains self-surveillance in order to avoid treatment for delinquency, mental illness or sexual perversity. As numerous forms of deviance were dealt with by the state, the necessity of the person to conform to behavioural patterns that demonstrated that one was normal became stronger. Connolly writes:

> The emergence of modern practices of bureaucratic control, market discipline, therapeutic help, democratic virtue, and sexual liberation, though each often defines itself in opposition to others, meshes with the global tendency of modern orders to organize the self into an agent of self-containment.
>
> (Connolly 1992: 150)

In terms of the argument presented in this volume, the panoptic structure also functions to break up face-to-face relations between subjects in order to strengthen their integration from 'above'. This is seen in the prohibition of speech in the classroom, the ideal of individual confinement of prisoners and the separation of factory workers. Disciplinary apparatuses thus foster a sense of individuality by addressing, or interpellating, subjects *as* individuals. A relationship between an individualized self and an institutionalized other thus comes to overlay and partly replace the relationship between a collectivized 'we' and 'they'.

The development of such institutionalized applications of expert knowledge was of course a central concern of classical social theory, and most nineteenth-century theorists were very aware of the conflict between coexisting traditional and emergent modern ways of life. Take Marx on the disciplinary conditions of the factory worker, for example. Both Marx and Foucault describe the increasingly cost-effective and intense control of the body in space and time geared to certain outputs, but they have different understandings of the subjectivity of the worker. While Marx sees workers' humanity (in a taken-for-granted sense) being destroyed by the alienation of their labour and the discipline that enforces it, Foucault's writing lacks any consideration of the prior ontological depth of the disciplined subject. This subject, as Marx noted in the case of work, is already constituted through a deeply embedded shared culture. Marx understood that the disciplines of the workplace continually clash with such localized, solidaristic and deeply held subjectivities (Marx 1976).

Foucault's followers are similarly quiet about the modes of embodiment that were in competition with the new medical 'fabrication' of the body. They are instead inclined to treat the rise of medical power as the beginning of the social constitution of embodiment, as if the constitution of embodiment were not a social process prior to the advent of this form of professional-institutional integration (Armstrong 1985). David Armstrong, attempting to explain to a sceptical sociological audience Foucault's claim that the body was 'fabricated' at the end of the eighteenth century, merely points to the beginnings of the medicalization of embodiment in this period, confusing an epistemological development with an ontological development.

Critiques of self-care promotion

Foucault's later work on governmentality, which focuses on these reflexive techniques of the self, has been drawn upon to critique the ways in which the state seeks to engender feelings of personal responsibility in citizens who then voluntarily participate in their own governance. Much of this writing draws on the work of Nikolas Rose, and, in particular, his influential book *Governing the Soul: the Shaping of the Private Self* (1990). Along with a number of other writers inspired by Foucault, Rose has theorized the ways in which 'governance', in its broadest sense, increasingly shapes the self-active capacities of autonomous individuals in order to instil desired behaviours. However, he sees the supposed autonomous self-identity of contemporary subjects as a fiction perpetrated by certain groups of intellectuals in order to support their professional or political power. Rose maintains that there is, in reality, nothing distinctively new about the contemporary forms of self-identity. He observes:

> Attempts to manage the enterprise to ensure productivity, competitiveness and innovation, to regulate child rearing to maximize emotional health and intellectual ability, to act upon dietary and other regimes in order to minimize disease and maximize health no longer seek to discipline, instruct,

moralize or threaten subjects into compliance. Rather they aspire to instil and use the self-directing propensities of subjects to bring them into alliance with the aspirations of authorities.

(Rose 1992: 153)

Rose has theorized the ways in which 'governance', in its broadest sense, increasingly shapes the self-active capacities of autonomous individuals in order to instil desired behaviours. Such poststructuralist theories provide many valuable insights into contemporary governmentality. However, they fail to set these strategies in the context of more concrete social changes and the changing patterns of social integration that are the structural preconditions for such governmental techniques. By confining themselves to an overly linguistic analysis, governmentality theorists see the contemporary emphasis on personal autonomy as merely a neo-liberal fiction, whereas I argue that such overblown accounts of personal agency are expressions of a real ontological condition that should not be ignored.

Rose sees the supposed autonomous self-identity of contemporary subjects as a fiction perpetrated by certain groups of intellectuals in order to support their professional or political power. He maintains that there is, in reality, nothing distinctively new about the contemporary forms of self-identity. Rose would dispute a sociological history of subjectivity that points to an increase in self-awareness and heightened sense of personal autonomy. Drawing on histories of private life, he points out that subjectivity was never simply a taken-for-granted, stable ontological foundation in pre-modern societies:

> ... from pagan Rome through Byzantium and onwards, in a multitude of different ways, the minutiae of the conduct of human beings has been attended to, described, judged, codified and instructed in relation to a whole range of practices, from those of domestic architecture to those of marital morality and sexual renunciation.

(Rose 1996: 303)

Rose is correct in pointing to the long history of professional-institutional integration, but he neglects at this point in his argument to discuss the relative importance of this level of integration as compared with the face-to-face. This is not to say that there was not a neat historical transformation from a taken-for-granted 'traditional' culture to a socially engineered 'modern' culture, but the governmentality theorists here overemphasize continuity while underestimating discontinuities. Drawing on studies of sexuality in early Christianity, Rose argues that 'there is nothing unprecedented about an intense problematization of the conduct of the self' (Rose 1996: 307). While such problematizations are not at all novel, what is novel, however, is not only the extent of such problematizations (dealing with more spheres of life and reaching the mass of the population rather than the most detraditionalized elites), but also the fact that such problematizations have become routinized and totally enmeshed with systems of expertise, wealth and power. In criticizing, quite rightly, the tendency to over-periodize such transformations, Rose is in danger of arguing that, with regard to the problematization of subjectivity, nothing changes apart from the content of the injunctions. In pointing out the existence of cultural diversity and plurality in pre-modern societies, Rose tends to argue that there is nothing different about the plurality of cultural forms and subject positions in contemporary Western societies. In conclusion he argues that

> the whole analytic of individualization is misplaced. It is not useful to oppose 'traditional' practices which problematize human beings in terms of allegiance – to a community, a lineage or a group – and 'modern' practices which problematize them in terms of individuality and autonomy.
>
> (Rose 1996: 309)

Rose suggests that if there appears to be certain sorts of subjects in certain historical spaces, this is not due to ontological changes, but is because 'different localized practices [...] presuppose, represent and act upon human beings as if they were persons of certain sorts' (Rose 1996: 312). That is, there is no difference in ontology, only a difference in the way people are described. At the same time, Rose argues against Rieff and Lasch's more pessimistic view of the erosion of meaningful social life and strong relationships, as elaborated in the previous chapter. He believes:

> The relations between psychotherapeutics and political power reveal not the devastation of the psychic autonomy and security of the self, but the fabrication of the autonomous self as the key term in analyses of social ills and cures, as the object of expert knowledge, as the target of systems of moral orthopaedics.
>
> (Rose 1990: 217)

Having argued that there is neither more nor less a sense of autonomy in the present, Rose goes on to claim that the allegedly more autonomous contemporary self-identity is a fiction created by psycho-technologists and others to legitimate their governmental technologies. (This approach has been widely applied to health promotion, and forms one of the major social scientific interpretations of the political dimensions of self-care, which I will return to below.) Rose points to the development of a scientistic 'authorization of authority' used by expert, professional and bureaucratic agencies to legitimate a new expertise of self-conduct. In this group he includes clinical medicine, psychiatry, criminology, psychology, statistics, pedagogy and sociology. These disciplines have entered into 'complex and contestatory relations' with other types of ethics maintained by theological, juridical and customary authorities and have combined to create a new realm of the social in which political strategies involved in the government of a polity are aligned with the regulation of the self-government of the citizen (Rose 1996: 317). Rose argues that the experience of a heightened sense of responsibility for one's self is not so much an ontological by-product of historical transformations as a deliberately cultivated and delusory belief. This ideology of autonomy allows for the penetration of power deeper into the person, while disguising this as the expansion of personal freedom. Rose points out that the valorization of 'autonomy, freedom, choice, authenticity, enterprise, lifestyle' has not developed innocently in an amorphous cultural space but instead operates as 'a grid of regulatory ideals' produced by various authorities, including doctors, managers and politicians. Many of the techniques upon which these 'new modalities for folding authority into the self' rely have been provided by the psycho-sciences (Rose 1996: 320–1).

I agree with Rose that an ideology of autonomy is promoted by those who use self-activating constitutive practices in order to emphasize the potentially liberating disembedding effects of more abstract levels of integration, while hiding the power which they wield. That is, people are only generally told how free they are when they are being encouraged to make a certain choice. The rise of psychotherapeutic expertise is itself a part of the broader structural changes in the integration of subjects, which fosters a perception of the loosening of restrictive ties and the expansion of choice. Power is not necessarily reaching any deeper into the person, but the more abstract constitutive practices facilitate a heightened self-consciousness and a more overt politicization of reflexive processes.

Rose goes on to discuss the effects of the media on self-consciousness, pointing out that the habitat of the modern subject is saturated with mediated images of self-conduct, self-formation and self-problematization. As well as the more obvious self-help or lifestyle programmes, news, drama and soap operas also illuminate life-decision and moral predicaments and 'presuppose certain repertoires of personhood as the *a priori* of the forms of life they display' (Rose 1996: 321). Rose tends to focus on the content of the electronic media – the types of people, types of problems, types of solutions, and the ways in which that content shapes subjectivity – without taking into account the formal features of the electronic media as a mode of social integration. Such an analysis of the message, which fails to take account of the nature of the medium, misses many of the ontological effects of the mass media and treats their content as mere stories. I am arguing that such an analysis of the effects of the media needs to look at the more fundamental effects of the dominance of the disembodied level of integration over the face-to-face and professional-institutional levels.

At this point, though, let us reflect on the relationship between the mass media and the medical profession. The recent rise of disembodied level of integration and the development of self-care promotion content has visibly undermined the authority of the medical profession, as with many other forms of professional-institutional power. This can be traced to the wider array of information available, and hence the popular awareness of differences of expert opinion and the desire to take a more active part in one's self-care, which has been encouraged in the media, but has been slow to be taken on board by professional health-care providers. These effects on the professional–patient relationship are of course influenced by the particular stories that are told in the media, but on a more general level, the relationship is profoundly altered by the mere existence of alternate sources of information irrespective of the specific content of that information.

Rose also overlooks the commodification of reflexive practices such as self-care. New techniques of risk calculation have allowed for the problematization of fields of experience and the production of risk-minimization techniques which are communicated to individuals in order to facilitate self-management (Rose 1996: 320). The marketing of goods and services uses the media to relate consumption and identity, and in the case of health, Rose observes that marketers 'establish a relation to their subjects that presupposes freedom, a freedom understood in terms of the wish of individuals to conduct their lives as projects for the minimization of risks and the maximization of quality of life' (Rose 1996: 321). He treats this ideology as a purely fictional construct perpetrated by advertisers. In fact, conducting one's life as a project of balancing competing risks and rewards is an inescapable part of everyday life for the consumer of self-care advice and any good or service with claimed health benefits or costs. Advertisers conceal the powers that shape our choices while making us think we are freer than we are, but this does not change the fact that the requirement to be a choosing subject is an intrinsic feature of commodification.

Deborah Lupton (1994, 1995) observes that because liberal democratic societies place limits on the power of the state to venture into people's lives, the government of subjectivity has to be carried out surreptitiously. Expertise

> achieves its effects not through threat of violence or constraint but by way of the persuasion inherent in its truths, the anxieties stimulated by its norms, and the attraction exercised by the images of life and self it offers to us.

The state (which is often equated with power) creates in its subjects the desires which it then acts to satisfy. Power aims to develop a symmetry between subjects' values and desires and its own political imperatives 'of consumption, profitability, efficiency, and social order' (Lupton 1995: 10). Lupton and Alan Petersen have developed a prolific critique of health promotion from this standpoint. While they provide a thorough elaboration of some of the political debates surrounding public health, they suffer from the same crude linguistic 'social constructionism' as Rose, in that they are concerned only with analysing public health as a set of discursive practices and tend to disregard the structural conditions which underlie the promotion of self-care. For example, in a discussion of the pervasiveness of the concept of 'risk', they begin by pointing out that risks are sociocultural constructs and go on to enumerate the political effects of the identification of health risks. While they are quick to point out that 'risk assessment has facilitated "government at a distance"', they gloss over the social preconditions which have made such risk assessments possible and desirable to governments, and as a consequence have a tendency to develop conspiracy theories in which political *effects* of specific forms of expertise are mistaken for *causal explanations* for the development of that knowledge in the first place (Petersen and Lupton 1996). I will discuss the development of individualized risk management in the next chapter, but in doing so, I believe it is necessary to look at the scientific techniques, the commercial motivations and the forms of communication which have made such risk management possible, rather than seeing it as a product of a particular political ideology.

The ideology of autonomy is not merely a fictitious interpretation of contemporary experience imposed by those with expertise in order to legitimate their power. It also reflects an ontological condition stemming from fundamental shifts in the dominant forms of social integration. To overlook the relationships between the form and content of these structural developments is to ignore the constitutive power of these more abstract forms of integration. In the next chapter I will discuss three features of late capitalist societies which shape the experience of personal autonomy and contribute to the belief that individuals determine their own health. At this point I want to explore the ways in which governmentality theorists relate a critique of autonomy to a critique of a neo-liberal ideology which expresses similar assumptions about the nature of the person.

Understanding neo-liberalism

Contemporary right-wing views on self-care have three defining features. Firstly, they retain a conservative concern with maintaining or resurrecting 'traditional' ways of life, values and institutions. Secondly, they espouse a radical individualism, which ironically serves further to undermine these traditional social forms by focusing on the 'empowerment' of autonomous individuals by integrating them more thoroughly in the market. Thirdly, the Right argues that the welfare state breeds dependency and saps people's motivation to actively care for themselves. The Right emphasizes the freedom of the individual to create their own circumstances, and in this it has much in common with individualistic self-help. Yet while much self-care advice stresses the dangers of passivity for individuals, neo-conservative social critics go further, seeing many of the social problems of modern societies as being caused by a pacified population, dependent on a paternalistic welfare state.

There is a libertarian strain on the Right who tend to argue against a large degree of state involvement in self-care promotion because of concerns about the state infringing on the free decision-making of individuals (Johnston and Ulyatt 1991). Such an approach would hold that the state has no place directing people not to engage in behaviour that may be a health risk to themselves but does not directly impinge on the rights of others. A Thatcher government MP expressed this difficulty during a 1980 parliamentary debate on a health promotion issue:

> How far are a government justified in taking action to seek to persuade people to abandon a course of conduct which that government believe to be

harmful? Particularly, should this question be asked of a Government who have been elected to reduce the interference of the State in the lives of the people and leave individuals greater freedom to make their own decisions?

(quoted in Leichter 1991: 82)

These libertarians have not been at all influential in shaping policy in conservative parties around the world, who have instead championed the criminalization of recreational drugs, euthanasia and various other forms of potential self-harm. Principles of individual freedom, while forming a central plank in the rhetoric of the Right, have been less important than the religious paternalism in which the state reasserts and rewards self-care practices which reflect a supposedly 'traditional morality'. The religious Right in the United States has, since the 1970s, been active in promulgating a conservative Christian ethics of self-care, which opposes illicit drug use, sexual promiscuity, abortion and the use of pornography, to name a few.

Religious paternalism is often justified on economic grounds, the logic being that un-Christian ways of living place an unacceptable strain on the public purse. New Right groups such as Empower America, a 'progressive-conservative' think-tank and lobby group in the United States, argue that the welfare state merely encourages 'irresponsible social behaviour'. Their solution to child poverty is to end state support for unwed mothers, creating the conditions in which 'young girls considering having a child out of wedlock would face more deterrents, greater social stigma and more economic penalties if they had babies' (Bennett 1996). This line of argument assumes that young women make rational decisions based on the costs and benefits of having a child, and that they then decide to have children because it will prove beneficial to them. The objection, often raised by supporters of welfare, that many of these pregnancies are the result of non-decisions, such as the absence or failure of contraception, rather than being actively planned, is not generally disputed. Empower America argues that these women should be forced to start making these decisions more consciously and actively rather than allowing themselves to be the passive victims of their circumstances. The poor need to be encouraged to be more self-active in maintaining their own welfare, rather than relying on the state to support them, they argue. While forcefully asserting the freedom of the individual, they insist that one's capacity for autonomous life-planning must be used responsibly. The decision to have a child out of wedlock is 'socially irresponsible', and the state should use all the forces at its disposal to ensure that women do not use their freedom 'irresponsibly'. They report that the Right in American politics is coming to see this as a moral issue: 'Having a child out-of-wedlock is wrong – not simply economically unwise for the individuals involved, or a financial burden on society, but morally wrong' (Bennett and Wehner 1996). This moral argument was launched by Empower America alongside unsourced, but apparently 'the most reliable', projections that, by the end of the 1990s, 40 per cent of all American births and 80 per cent of minority births would be out-of-wedlock. In fact, in 2000, around 31 per cent of all births in the United States were to women out of wedlock. The rate was lower for Hispanic women (30 per cent) and White non-Hispanic women (26 per cent), but higher for Black women (62 per cent). A very high proportion of teenage mothers (83 per cent) are umarried (Bachu and O'Connell 2001: 5). By exaggerating these figures and failing to take into account the underlying socio-economic causes of this situation, the message to the poor and minority groups is that their poverty, rather than being an entrenched structural feature of American society, is a result of their own immoral actions.

In the United States, the New Right's various moral crusades – including those against welfare spending, abortion and homosexuality – are all seen as battles against 'permissiveness'. John Knowles (1977a, 1977b), then president of the Rockefeller Foundation, used the editorial column of *Science* to explain that health maintenance requires the very qualities – self-discipline and restraint – being undermined by the permissive society:

> Prevention of disease means forsaking the bad habits which many people enjoy – overeating, too much drinking, taking pills, staying up at night, engaging in promiscuous sex, driving too fast, and smoking cigarettes – or put another way, it means doing the things that require special effort – exercising regularly, improving nutrition, going to the dentist, practicing contraception, ensuring harmonious family life, submitting to screening examinations.
>
> (Knowles 1977a: 1103)

Up to the late 1960s the term 'permissiveness' was rarely used outside of discussions of child-rearing practices, but from the late 1960s it was used disparagingly to describe sexual freedoms and then, later, social policies and views which were seen as indulgent (Thomas 1969). New Right writers argue that a lack of discipline in a child's upbringing results in a licentiousness and lack of self-discipline in adulthood which is the root cause of sexual promiscuity and drug use. And since virtually all social ills are attributed to sex and drugs by the New Right, it is this lack of self-discipline which needs be addressed by the state and New Right social movements. In this way, the New Right is a key player in reducing contemporary social problems to issues of individual decision-making, which drastically overemphasize the freedom of the individual to create their own social conditions.

It is ironic that the New Right seeks to activate individuals by highlighting and heightening their status as self-serving consumers in the postmodern market. The central feature of New Right welfare reforms is a move to an 'incentive-oriented' form of welfare based on 'the incentives of the market, the urgency of virtue, and the desire of all people to improve their lot in life' (Empower America 1996). As I argued earlier in this volume, I agree with the New Right that the market is indeed powerful in constituting such a self-active form of subjectivity. What they fail to realize, however, is that the relentless expansion of the market into the private sphere, which they seek to speed up, is a major element in the 'hedonistic' culture they are critical of. On a broad level, the market encourages an individualized preoccupation with the satisfaction of one's every desire. If we look more specifically at the New Right's preoccupation with sex and drugs, it is obvious that both sexuality and drug use have been thoroughly commodified. The New Right's restrictions on market exchange in these specific areas is an authoritarian restriction on the freedom of both producers and consumers which causes considerable tensions between the libertarian and conservative groupings on the Right.

Within New Right commentaries on self-care, there is an overt awareness of the state's power to constitute subjectivity, not merely seeing it as a restriction of freedom, as classical liberalism was inclined to do. Early liberalism was more inclined to treat the market in a more taken-for-granted sense, seeing it as a natural feature of human societies, compared with the more common neo-liberal understanding of the market as an 'artificial' entity which must be actively created (Burchell 1996: 270–1). Because of neo-liberalism's desire to reconstruct the dominant culture away from the passive dependence allegedly instilled by the welfare state, neo-liberalism is more favourably disposed towards using the state in a constitutive manner than was classical liberalism. In relation to the market, there is a similar belief that the state, having distorted the natural market for so long, must be actively engaged in constructing the free market anew.

Against welfarist models of government, neo-liberalism promotes an enterprise culture which is centred on a set of virtues including competitive striving, boldness and vigour. These are tied to a politics which aims to enhance individual freedom through the maximization of choice directed to self-fulfilment. As Rose and others have pointed out, both neo-liberal ethics and the therapeutic domain presuppose the 'autonomization' and 'responsibilization' of the self. In both these fields of discourse, Rose says,

> the individual is to become, as it were, an entrepreneur of itself, seeking to maximize its own powers, its own happiness, its own quality of life, through enhancing its autonomy and then instrumentalizing its autonomous choices in the service of its own lifestyle.
>
> (Rose 1992: 150–1)

Neo-liberalism and therapeutic cultures are thus both inclined to conceive of social well-being in individualistic and psychologistic ways, as a reflection of successful or unsuccessful self-management. In this view, work on the self (through exercise, therapy or eating habits, etc.) has the capacity to enhance not only health and happiness, but also one's socio-economic status. Blockages in the process of active self-constitution – especially negativity and passivity – are therefore blamed as the major impediments to well-being, trapping people in powerless and dependent situations.

Rose's political point is that 'in embracing such an ethic of psychological health construed in terms of autonomy, we are condemned to make a project out of our own identity and we have become bound to the powers of expertise' (Rose 1992: 153). My objection is not with his quite accurate assessment of expert power, but with his assessment of the merely ideological nature of such ethics, which ignores the real conditions to which such ethics respond. It is clear that in a system which presupposes and encourages self-active life planning on so many levels, it is a precondition of effective action that one make a 'project' of one's life. Rather than being purely rhetorical devices, the psychological and cultural ideals proposed by neo-liberalism represent a normative set of strategies for negotiating late or postmodern social structures. These 'ideals' acknowledge contemporary reality – faced with the structural requirement to be a choosing subject, the refusal or inability to choose leads quickly to social redundancy. Although the options available are of course highly circumscribed, this require-ment that we choose emanates from all institutions we deal with. Schools require that students choose subjects and career paths well before they have the experi-ence which could let them know what career they want. Advertising reminds us that we must constantly choose our clothes, our food, our medicines and our preferred form of exercise. I am trying here not to legitimate the neo-liberal response, but only to argue that any persuasive critique of such 'consumerist' ethics must acknowledge the ontological condition to which they appeal, and seek to formulate a less socially destructive response to these conditions drawing on more socially empathic and cooperative values.

Neo-liberal government involves the use by the state of activating technolo-gies developed in various spheres. As the earlier rise of the disciplinary state involved the adoption by the state of governmental techniques developed in the then-emergent modern institutions, the current shift involves a reorientation of state activity in line with techniques of government being developed by contem-porary institutions that use the power of disembodied integration. As Rose and Miller have observed, rather than an overall reduction in the level of state inter-vention, neo-liberalism represents 'a re-organization of political rationalities that brings them into a kind of alignment with contemporary technologies of govern-ment' (Rose and Miller 1992: 199). The welfare state set about building 'social' solutions, aiming to create the structural conditions whereby all could feel secure. Public health, before the shift to a lifestyle-oriented health promotion, used professionals and expertise in general to improve primarily the conditions of life, thereby maximizing the health of a population. Advanced liberal or neo-liberal rule, Rose points out,

> depends upon expertise in a different way, and articulates experts differently into the apparatus of rule. It does not seek to govern through 'society', but through the regulated choices of individual citizens. And it seeks to detach the substantive authority of expertise from the apparatus of political rule, relocating experts within a market governed by the rationalities of competi-tion, accountability and consumer demand.
>
> (Rose 1993: 285)

This marketization is understood as a process of autonomization of society in as much as the increasing integration into the market increases autonomy with regard to the state and competing social and political logics (Burchell 1996).

Unlike most contemporary political theory, the governmentality theorists have recognized that one of the most significant features of neo-liberalism is that through its philosophy the Right 'succeeded in formulating a political rationality consonant with the new regime of the self' (Rose 1992: 160). While the Left has been divided over the increasing individualization of contemporary social life, the Right has been able to produce a political language which resonates with the active self-identity which has accompanied these technologies. That is, while the Left has been sceptical, for good reason, of the popular desire for the expansion of 'choice', on the one hand, and the psychologization of social issues, on the other, the Right has been effective in formulating a radically new political philosophy which is able to celebrate these experiences, while at the same time forging a sense of continuity with classical liberal, and even conservative, philosophies.

In relation to self-care, Rose and Miller refer to the activation of patients in relation to their health as leading to the emergence of a 'neo-liberal' mode of government of health. 'The patient', they observe, was 'to be actively enrolled in the government of health, educated and persuaded to exercise a continual informed scrutiny of the health consequences of diet, lifestyle and work' (Rose and Miller 1992: 195). While it is true that a neo-liberalist response to these self-activating developments in health has been extremely influential, Rose and Miller tend to collapse together therapeutic techniques and the political responses to them, seeing a neo-liberalist ethic inherent within the self-care orientation from the beginning: 'Out of this concatenation of programmes, strategies and resistances, a new "neo-liberal" mode of government of health was to take shape' (Rose and Miller 1992: 195). Rose and Miller tend to see in the rise of self-care a therapeutic orientation that leads necessarily to a political expression in the form of neo-liberal philosophies. It should be remembered, though, that self-care models have been employed and celebrated within very different political camps. Self-help groups, for example, vary widely in their political stances, and the political potential of such groups has been trumpeted both by the women's movement and by economic rationalist health service planners who desire a shift from professional to less expensive voluntary service provision. Feminist groups in the 1970s saw the self-help form of organization used in consciousness-raising groups as a means of undermining patriarchal organizational forms and of creating an empowering space for the sharing of experiences. Conversely, the employment of self-help for cost reduction may fit neatly into a broader neo-liberal approach to government, but this does not mean that self-help is necessarily aright-wing form of health care.

While Rose and Miller provide an illuminating assessment of the neo-liberal enterprise culture and the subjectivity that underlies it, they focus on the content of health messages while ignoring the changes in the form of transmission of self-care knowledge and practices. Consequently, their analysis is limited because it treats the neo-liberal appeal to consumer freedom as mere political rhetoric.

By confining themselves to an overly linguistic analysis, governmentality theorists tend to see the contemporary emphasis on self-care as simply a neo-liberal fiction. I argue that the desire for personal autonomy, which neo-liberals exploit for political purposes, is a more pervasive feature of contemporary Western societies, and not merely political rhetoric. This experience of self-active subjectivity is a real condition of contemporary life and neo-liberalism has been much more adept at incorporating that experience into a political ideology than has the Left.

The ontological dimension to the New Right's victim-blaming is rarely discussed. As Zygmunt Bauman has argued, in postmodern societies there is a section of the population who are excluded by poverty from the 'consumer freedom' experienced by the bulk of the population. In a society of 'free consumers' the poor are socially defined as flawed consumers whose 'imperfection', he says, 'consists in their inability to enter the free-choice game, in their ostensible incapacity to exercise their individual freedom and conduct their life-business as a private matter between them and the market' (Bauman 1988: 84). The 'consuming classes' understand their level of consumer freedom as a pay-off for personal striving, self-discipline and endurance in the comparatively 'un-free' realm of work. Personal success or failure is increasingly individualized as the result of such personal qualities and strivings. To many of these 'self-made' members of the consuming class, the poor appear as lazy or incompetent individuals rather than as unfortunate victims of their circumstances, as was the implicit understanding legitimizing the welfare state.

The New Right fuels such individualistic understandings of poverty by promoting the view that the unemployed simply lack motivation and self-discipline. It encourages a distinction between an unmotivated, 'undeserving poor' who lack initiative and an entrepreneurial deserving poor who are willing to subject themselves to the most oppressive working conditions yet have little freedom in the market (Bessant 1994). Those who have shown an inability to discipline themselves in order to participate in the consumer society are subjected to the panoptic discipline of an increasingly repressive welfare state and at the same time are subjected to training courses, case-managers and seminars designed to inculcate them with the self-direction required in the workforce (McDonald 1993). The New Right's political rhetoric abrogates any collective responsibility for the poor, who are cast as irresponsible burdens on tax-payers. The consumer class's desire for higher disposable incomes and fewer restrictions on their consumer freedom is achieved by shrinking the welfare state and the further immiseration and repression of those whose heteronomous conditions prevent them from exercising the freedom and autonomy others enjoy. Meanwhile, the structural and political causes of unemployment and inequality are virtually ignored. Neo-liberal economic policies have the effect of widening economic inequalities, which in turn causes greater differentials in health status, and the privatization of social and health-care services further restricts access to the poor.

9 Reflexivity, rationalization and health risks

Are you at health-risk? A lifestyle inventory provides information on your present state of health, and creates a personalized report for you which focuses on lifestyle practices you can change to improve the quality of your life.

How healthy is your diet? Now you can find out with a computerized program that informs you on what percent of your diet is fats, proteins, carbohydrates and your R.D.A. for vitamins, minerals and water.

Website of the Exercise Science, Fitness and Lifestyle Assessment Centre at Canada's Malaspina University College, 1998

Lifestyle assessments provide individuals with expert advice to guide the conduct of everyday life, including a systematic inventory of current practices, an identification of risks and recommended self-care strategies to minimize such risks and improve well-being. This chapter looks at the cultural implications of such rationalization of self-care practices, through an analysis of the work of Anthony Giddens, Ulrich Beck and others. It concentrates on the contemporary production of biomedically framed health risks by expert systems. While their organization and methods of inquiry differ dramatically, all of these expert systems have in common a more or less systematic body of knowledge that is relatively inaccessible to lay people. I look at the ways in which risk anxiety is selectively heightened or alleviated in order to bring about behaviour change.

The dominant mode of inquiry in contemporary Western societies, which I will refer to as 'technoscientific', overlays and reconstitutes less systematically produced culturally based forms of knowledge. I have alluded to tensions between technoscientific and 'folk', 'lay' or 'informally culturally reproduced' forms of knowledge, but in this chapter I will concentrate on the effects of the contemporary production of biomedically framed health risks. I will use the term 'expert system' to refer to systematic and institutionalized bodies of knowledge produced by intellectually trained specialists. This term is broad enough to encompass scientific health research as well as the numerous 'alternative' systems that are prominent in producing self-care knowledge, such as naturopathy and chiropractic. While their organization and methods of inquiry differ dramatically, all of these expert systems have in common a more or less systematic body of knowledge that is relatively inaccessible to lay people.

Expert systems are based on impersonal principles that exist independently of the individual practitioner and the specific context in which the expertise is applied. In relation to the social contexts in which they are applied, modern expert systems tend to evacuate local and culturally specific content and replace it with a more organized body of knowledge which extends across broad time-space bands (Giddens 1994b: 84–5). The practitioners are to an extent interchangeable, given competence in a body of knowledge: experts reassure their lay clients by advertising their possession of interchangeable institutional knowledge; doctors display their degrees on the walls of their consulting rooms; while authors list their credentials on the back cover of self-help books.

Since their inception, the biosciences have been employed by those institutions that sought to shape the behaviour of populations, and this integration of psychology, epidemiology, architecture and numerous other human sciences with systems of control has been well documented by Foucault and many of the other theorists discussed above. These tended to act upon the subject unconsciously through contextual means, or at least without their active cooperation. Here I am interested in the more recent application of these and other expert systems to produce self-care techniques which are employed reflexively by self-active subjects. Most self-care techniques are means of avoiding identified health risks, and in the section below I want to explore the way in which such risks are identified and communicated to the public.

It is useful to begin by distinguishing between traditional and modern hazards (Giddens 1990: 109–11). In traditional societies, few hazards could be predicted and controlled, whereas in modern societies many of the hazards that plagued traditional societies have been brought under human control. The status of these hazards was in the process transformed from unpredictable 'acts of God' to knowable 'risks' which were able to be more clearly identified, calculated and managed by expert systems. The expansion and development of science and rational organization was expected to create societies in which knowledge became increasingly certain and control increasingly effective. Medicine, as part of this endeavour, has sought to beat these threats (diseases) by finding 'cures' for each in turn. This fantasy of the eventual 'control' of health and illness was not challenged by public health, which showed by the 1970s that many of the threats to health were not of biological origin, but of social origin. The dream of identification and control was simply extended to the social realm – and the task of understanding and controlling the social determinants of disease became a new field of inquiry and intervention.

To a significant extent, modern societies have created major areas of life which are relatively safe, secure and predictable. However, alongside these areas of security, they contain areas of profound doubts and insecurities. Some of these insecurities are vestiges of traditional hazards which have not yet been adequately understood and controlled by science, such as muscular dystrophy or earthquakes. But new and relatively unforeseen risks have emerged which have been created by modernization itself. The Enlightenment project of control over nature and society leads to certainties and predictability in some areas of life, but also has the capacity to produce uncertainties on a scale never before humanly possible, such as global warming or the possibility of nuclear war.

Ulrich Beck, the most prominent sociological writer on risk, uses the term to refer only to the hazards produced by modernization. In contrast to older dangers, Beck defines the concept of risk as a 'systematic way of dealing with hazards and insecurities induced and introduced by modernity itself' (Beck 1992: 21). Beck's analysis centres on the fact that contemporary societies are forced to confront the 'latent side-effects' of modernization, arguing that the invisible risks produced by the system are nearing the end of their latency (Beck 1992: 55). By using the term 'risk society', Beck is describing a stage of modernity in which the threats produced by modernization itself come to predominate, and the distribution of these risks (the distribution of bads rather than goods) becomes increasingly important politically (Beck 1994). Whereas politics in industrial societies is centred on distribution of goods, politics in risk societies is more concerned with the distribution of 'bads'.

Here I am concerned with two types of *abstract risks*: the first are those modernization risks described by Beck and others; the second are those risks which predate modernization but which are able to be identified much more precisely with the aid of abstract forms of inquiry. Take alcohol consumption, for example. Every society in which alcohol is consumed has theories about the positive and negative effects of alcohol consumption, and until recently these understandings were usually based on generations of accumulated experience and observation. In recent decades there have been mountains of statistical evidence describing the health effects of alcohol consumption, which is communicated to the population in order to shape their drinking habits. Regardless of the fact that the statistical information is inconclusive and the expert advice seems to change every few years, the fact remains that the way the public perceives the health effects of drinking has been gradually transformed. The dangers of alcohol are not produced by modernization, but our understanding of those dangers in terms of abstract risks is a feature of highly detraditionalized societies. I will treat these expertly defined natural hazards as abstract risks in as much as they are identified, communicated and managed by expert systems in the modern era. Beck assumes that all the risks identified by science are themselves the products of science, which is clearly not the case. Take, for example, the speculated increased risk of cancer caused by eating charred foods. An identifiable risk is created by an abstract mode of inquiry delving into an aspect of life which had never been considered a hazard. But it is wrong to blame nutritionists and oncologists for producing the risk. It is true, of course, that the risk they identify may be purely imaginary, but it is also possible that the hazard has existed all along and has only now been identified.

New forms of expertise have developed since the late twentieth century which have greatly expanded the capacity to predict the health consequences of individuals' lifestyles, and derive more detailed calculations of risk, and predict effects further into the person's future. This is in part due to the development of a more finely tuned art of statistical correlation which has been made possible by computerized data collection and analysis (Finerman and Bennett 1995). Risk calculation usually leads to the production of risk-minimization techniques which are communicated to individuals in order to facilitate self-management. That is, in the contemporary period there is a much closer relationship between research and behaviour modification as a result of this precision. Even the 'alternative' forms of self-care generally base their risk assessments on scientifically defined risks to some extent, although the self-care techniques they advocate as risk-minimization strategies may not be endorsed by the scientific community. Vitamin therapies are an example of this, as are the currently popular techniques to combat free-radicals by ingesting anti-oxidants.

The fine tuning of scientific risk calculation does not only concern itself with behavioural practices, though, often identifying environmental risks which are not amenable to individualized risk minimization, such as the risks posed by urban air pollution. It is in these areas, where individuals do not have the option of a low-risk, low-anxiety behavioural alternative, that political challenges most often develop. Beck (1992) goes so far as to argue that in risk societies, solidarity is more often the result of shared anxiety than shared experiences of oppression or deprivation. One of the factors which draws people to the green movement, for example, is a heightened awareness of, and anxiety over, the health risks posed by environmental degradation. The social movements which are oriented towards the reduction of contextual risks are heavily middle-class in composition. The poor are unable to overcome individualized risks to the same extent as the wealthy, so their primary interest is in acquiring the resources necessary to reduce those individualized risks. The wealthy have the resources to be able to overcome individualized risks, but are frustrated by their inability to overcome shared contextual risks. As Bauman has noted,

> only such dangers from which the majority would see no political escape (that is, no chance of redistributing the risks to the weaker agents' households, or of purchasing risk-exemptions singly or severally) have a good chance to be universally noted by political actors and give birth to a truly unified and effective political action.
>
> (Bauman 1993: 208)

The risks from which there is no possibility of escape for the powerful are politicized. Where there is a behavioural means of risk minimization, the issue tends to be depoliticized, with the onus of action resting on the individual, regardless of the cause of the risk. Bryan Turner concludes that

> the way risk management has been institutionalised in consumer society allows the deployment of the reflexivity not so much as an instrument of individual freedom, fate-control, or colonisation of the future as a device to reforge public anxiety into corporate profits and, on the way, to further deflect public concerns away from the danger-perpetuating mechanism itself.
>
> (Turner 1994: 27)

I am suggesting that this is the case because most risk management techniques are developed and promoted by the private sector, and the producers of such techniques are interested only in selling their product and have little reason to become involved in tackling the causes of the risk. In such situations, producers will employ expert opinions selectively in order to convince consumers that a risk exists and that their product can minimize this risk. In marketing the product, little is said about other means of minimizing the risks because the consumer must be convinced that purchasing the product being advertised is the best form of protection.

For example, a company advertising sunscreen is likely to make reference to the depletion of the ozone layer as a cause of increased risk of skin cancer, but they are unlikely to use their advertising airtime telling people how the ozone layer can be regenerated. Thus the commodification of self-care practices leads the mass media and expert knowledge to be used in such a way as to place responsibility on individuals to employ individualized self-care practices in order to respond to systemically produced risks. Postmodernist writers on public health tend to see this focus on individualized health risk minimization as an effect of neo-liberal ideology (Petersen 1996). I hope to have shown here that the emphasis on personal responsibility is an outcome of structured social practices, not neo-liberal rhetoric.

The commonsensical distinction between healthy and unhealthy lifestyles is being eroded by the realization that every person engages in behaviours that carry health risks. An emphasis on the prevention of illness has involved a shift of the focus of interventions from actual illness to potential illness as the target of health-care intervention (Hughes 1994; Petersen 1996). Lifestyle surveys establish correlations between ever more subtle aspects of behaviour and health outcomes, and almost every aspect of life can be related to differentials in health outcomes. As the task of identifying all correlations between disparate behaviours and outcomes proceeds, the number of known health risks multiplies. And with the expansion of known risks, the scope of reflexive risk management further increases. Castel sees in this expansion of health risk minimization a situation in which

> [a] vast hygienist utopia plays on the alternate registers of fear and security, inducing a delirium of rationality, an absolute reign of calculative reason and a no less absolute prerogative of its agents, planners and technocrats, administrators of happiness for a life to which nothing happens.
>
> (Castel 1991: 289)

The modern ideologies of illness prevention are imbued with a grandiose technocratic rationalizing dream which aspires to absolute control over the accidental. This situation appears more bleak when Castel's observations, which relate primarily to collective risk minimization, are extrapolated to individualized risk minimization. Individual lifestyle choices are increasingly being treated as instrumental goal-directed strategies by health promotion agencies.

Lifestyle is itself transformed from a way of life based on tradition, ritual and commonsense in the direction of an idealized self-controlled way of living which is obsessed with the health consequences of every action, no matter how distant or immeasurable the effects. An abstracted lifestyle is consciously organized and directed at perfect health, which has become an end in itself. It is this elevation of health to an end in itself that the critics of narcissism criticize as an unfortunate obsession with the self. Self-care practices increasingly take the form of purposive-rational action (Habermas 1987: 336) in which participants are primarily interested in the consequences of their actions.

Habermas is useful here in elaborating the broader processes within which an instrumental orientation to self-care is located. He is critical of those, such as Weber, Adorno and Horkheimer, who describe the relentless expansion of instrumental reason. According to Habermas, they suggest 'that the rationality of knowing and acting subjects is systematically expanded into a purposive rationality of a higher order' (Habermas 1987: 333). In arguing that society is becoming increasingly rationalized, they confuse the rationalization of the system with the rationalization of action and they fail to recognize that action is also heavily shaped by a communicative rationality which stems from the lifeworld. Because they fail to take account of communicative rationality, the conventional rationalization thesis can only conceive of opposition to this systemic rationalization emanating from the power of the irrational, in the form of the charismatic power of the leader or in the mimetic power of art and love.

In health care the popularity of alternative and 'natural' health care movements can be seen to be in large part due to their promotion of themselves as more 'human' and 'natural' alternatives to the highly rationalized and technologized medical mainstream. This is undoubtedly true, but the other against which the rationalization of self-care is generally opposed is the realm of traditional self-care, which evolved and was expressed through the lifeworld. To use the example of sexual practices, although rationalized religious institutions have made pronouncements on sex for centuries, these usually took the form of prohibitions of certain practices rather than attempting to influence how sex was practised between couples. Foucault examines early phases in the development of productive power over sexuality, but the cultural manifestations of such forms of expertise have been much more readily apparent since the late twentieth century (Foucault 1981). Since the 1960s, a huge body of expertise has been developed which is routinely translated into advice for consumers in the form of magazine articles, psychotherapy and the array of goods and services produced by the sex industry. Sexual relations, once reconstituted with reference to this expertise, can be thought of as an increasingly systematized lifeworld.

This simple distinction between system and lifeworld begins to break down when we consider new social movements, in this case the natural health movement or the New Age movement. Habermas (1981) generally sees new social movements as acting to defend the lifeworld against colonization by the system. New social movements typically respond to systemic penetration of the lifeworld not by trying to shore up a pre-existing configuration, but with innovative alternatives which are only partially defensive of the lifeworld and which are usually highly integrated into the system in some way. Habermas makes an exception of feminism on these grounds, because feminism, he recognizes, is reacting against the systemic constitution of gender not by shoring up a traditional form but by reforming the 'grammar of forms of life'. Habermas's overly reactive model does not fit with most social movements, I would suggest, apart from the purely reactive conservative movements which hark back to 'traditional' values and ways of life. Like feminism, gay and lesbian movements and the green movement, to name a few, the self-help 'movement' in health care is not simply resistant to the abstraction of the realm of 'cultural reproduction, social integration, and socialization' (to use Habermas' terms). In health, the self-help movement has not simply reacted against medicalization in favour of an alternative already existing within the lifeworld; it creates an altogether different form which appeals to those disaffected by the abstraction of health care, but which is itself no less abstract.

There are interesting parallels between Beck's (1992) theoretical analysis and the natural health-care movement in their identification of the causes of health risks. Let me posit very crudely that orthodox medicine generally sees disease as a natural phenomenon which can be combated by science, or as a result of individual neglect which has allowed the body to succumb to natural degradation. The natural health-care movement, on the other hand, tends to see 'modern life' or technologization of life away from a 'natural' state as responsible for the majority of ailments. Often the immune system is cast as the body's own defence against the evils of civilization and technoscience. Beck falls into a similarly simplistic analysis, blaming science for all the threats to which people are subject in modern societies. For believers in natural health care, anxiety/risk can be alleviated by avoiding harmful invasions of the body by technoscience. Leading a 'natural' lifestyle is proposed as a way of minimizing the risks posed by life in late capitalism. This extends to avoiding 'invasive' treatments in which the integrity of the body is penetrated by technology (surgery, x-rays) and by avoiding the intake of the products of technoscience (pharmaceuticals, chemicals in food and water).

Packaging expertise

In drawing this distinction between experts and the lay population, it is important not to overlook the role of the 'intermediaries' who translate expert knowledge into popularly accessible information (Lidskog 1996). In face-to-face interactions between experts and non-experts, such as the case of the medical consultation, the expert is also the representative of an extensive expert system, in this case built around biomedical research. However, an increasingly significant proportion of self-care advice is communicated through print and electronic media by intermediaries such as journalists and scriptwriters, who are not experts themselves, but interpret expert knowledge and 'repackage' it for lay audiences. The types of people involved in this translation process are intellectual workers who can bridge the divide between the esoteric worlds of expert knowledge production and the cultural forms in which the information must be framed to ensure its accessibility by a lay audience. These intermediaries inevitably reframe the expert knowledge in light of their own institutional goals and take advantage of the heterogeneity of expert systems to produce advice that will sell, or sell a product or convince the audience to behave differently, depending on their particular commercial or governmental interests. It is possible to draw a distinction between those approaches that seek to instruct and those that seek to empower the audience. Mary Dixon-Woods' (2001) analysis of literature on how to communicate with patients using information leaflets reveals that what she calls the 'patient education discourse' predominates in published papers. The characteristics she includes in this category are: an interest in outcomes that have been defined as useful from a biomedical perspective; an assumption of patient incompetence; use of a mechanistic model of communication; a concern with defining and measuring quality; and a failure to engage with sociological criticisms of the biomedical model. She contrasts this approach with a 'patient empowerment discourse', which is both more recent and more scarce in published papers on how to use patient information leaflets. This approach is usually motivated by a patient-centred consumer advocacy agenda and commonly draws on sociological understandings of health and illness and a wider range of understandings of patients than biomedical approaches (Dixon-Woods 2001: 1419). The patient empowerment approach to health communications presumes that the reader is an active decision-maker and seeks to provide information to assist these choices, rather than assuming that patients' interests coincide with those of professionals.

A quick glance at the range of self-help books in any bookstore reveals a wide range of claims to authority and means of engaging readers. While some texts rely on the author's professional expertise (often signalled by the prominent placing of a 'PhD' or 'MD' on the cover), others written by informed non-experts are overtly subjective in their claims. These relatively non-authoritative self-care strategies are presented as helpful advice or things to try, usually with a disclaimer that the effectiveness and relevance of these tips can only be judged by the individual reader. Most contemporary self-help books seek to overcome the abstract distant relationship between author and reader by adopting a warm and familiar authorial tone, employing a level of intimacy that belies the anonymity of the textual encounter. The author seems to be saying, as Arlie Russel Hochschild has paraphrased, 'You and I, we are on our own – here's what I did. Why don't you try.' The author claims to know the reader by virtue of having been in the same situation and confides their innermost feelings to the reader in order to create the appearance of a meaningful sharing of information (Hochschild 1994: 6–7).

Most self-help books and commodified health advice presented in other media draw together snippets of information from an eclectic array of sources, including scientific knowledge, accepted popular wisdom gathered together by the author, and reflections drawn from personal experience. Dale Carnegie summed up this popular approach in the preface to his 1948 book, *How to Stop Worrying and Start Living*: ' "Science", said the French philosopher Valéry, "is a collection of successful recipes." That is what this book is, a collection of successful and time-tested recipes to rid our lives of worrying' (Carnegie 1962: xv). Carnegie was one of the high-fliers of mid-century American self-help and a pioneer in the genre. His YMCA courses began with public speaking but soon developed into teaching groups of keen-to-learn adult students how to win friends and influence people. Unable to find a suitable (suitably instrumental, he means) textbook on such 'human relations', he wrote one which sold a huge number, thereby launching his publishing career. A few years later Carnegie realized that 'another one of the biggest problems of these adults was worry' (Carnegie 1962: xvi), so he launched a new YMCA course on how to stop worrying, which led to another book. Carnegie considers teaching a helping profession, involved primarily with helping people to overcome their inner limitations, many of which, he believes, are caused by negative attitudes. He asked his students to implement a set of rules or techniques to manage their negative thoughts, which the students were then asked to evaluate for the class, along with other techniques they had found effective in the past. Using this process of distillation, Carnegie argues that he was able to use his teaching as a method of experimentation to ascertain which techniques were most effective and then reproduce them for the reading masses (Carnegie 1962: xv). This is not, then, 'poppsychology' (the popularization of an expert knowledge) but a distillation of lay knowledge and practices through anecdote, clichés and popular wisdom which is benevolent on the surface, but underneath is motivated by the desire for personal wealth on the part of both author and reader. In this regard Carnegie expresses a very instrumental attitude towards one's personality, which is evident in much self-help literature, encouraging the modification of any aspects of one's personality which seem incompatible with the needs of one's social and occupational circumstances. This readiness to re-create one's self is in stark contrast to a lack of interest in the broader social context of the person. This type of psychologistic self-help often focuses on cognition as if it is an internal process, so that when Carnegie says that 'worry is one of the biggest problems facing mankind' (Carnegie 1962: xv), he means that the prevalence of faulty cognitive processes is detrimentally affecting the collective health of humanity. By not even addressing the causes of worry, Carnegie implies that people have nothing legitimate to worry about. This sentiment reached its zenith in the middle of the Reagan era in the pop song 'Don't worry, be happy'. Carnegie seemed to believe that telling the masses how not to worry could dramatically improve the health of the nation. 'More than half our hospital beds', he states, 'are occupied by people with nervous and emotional troubles' (Carnegie 1962: xiv). As well as being gifted in synthesizing popular self-care techniques, Carnegie was conscious of the need to motivate his audience so that they would stick with his programme for self-transformation. He observed of his teaching days, 'I *had to motivate* my students. I *had* to help them *solve their problems*. I *had* to *make each session so inspiring that they wanted to continue coming*' (Carnegie 1962: xiii). Carnegie's books are some of the first examples of self-help books which aim to help the audience actively shore up their psychological integrity and actively build their own self-confidence (and therefore success, being the underlying promise).

Health-care professionals dispensing mediated health advice are often subject to institutionalized codes of conduct designed to ensure that they do not undermine or sully the reputation of the established body of expert knowledge held by that profession. To take the case of psychology as an example, experts with psychological training are now widely employed in the media, as experts on news programmes, as in-depth interviewers, as advisers to television and film writers, as writers of popular books and magazine articles, as visiting experts on chat shows and as personal advisers via 'talk-back' radio and magazine 'agony aunt' columns. At the same time as the self-help publishing explosion, 'talk-back' or 'call-in' radio programmes focusing on mental health and relationship themes started to appear in the early 1970s in the United States and soon after in Australia and Britain. Psychologists working in radio and television at the time were contravening the American Psychologists Association Code of Ethics, which prohibited giving 'personalized advice' via 'radio or television programs'. In response to the number and popularity of such programmes, the Association revised its code to recommend that '[w]hen personal advice is given by means of [...] radio or television programs [...] the psychologist utilizes the most current relevant data and exercises the highest level of professional judgement' (Bouhoutsos *et al.* 1986: 409). This allowed for open discussion of media psychology in a professional forum. Up to that time, most radio and television psychologists had effectively been self-taught, experimenting with styles and formats in an *ad hoc* fashion, but with the legitimation of the use of the mass media, a loose process of peer review and collaboration began in the psychological community. The rise of self-care advice in the media has widely challenged the authority of professionals in private consultation, but professionals are increasingly using the media in order to try to lift the public profile of their profession and its body of expert knowledge.

In order to overcome the chasm between the expert knowledge of health-care professionals and the situated experience of patients, a reflexivity is required on the part of both the practitioner and the patient. Earlier I discussed such efforts in medicine to introduce a more participatory role for the patient so that a dialogue can occur between the lay person and the expert. This requires a reflexivity on the part of the professional, who needs to understand the means of inquiry which inform their practice so that they can be aware of how the abstraction involved in biomedical inquiry affects they way they construct embodied conditions. That is, the dissection of the body, mental states and practices into discrete units for the purposes of study, and the development of highly abstract relationships between such units in expert systems, produces a very powerful body of knowledge, but one which is often meaningless to the person who is the object of such inquiry. This chasm is of crucial importance in the development of lifestyle advice, as biomedical categories often bear little relationship with the cultural categories which inform people's decision-making.

Consider, for example, the following excerpt from an analysis of the eating patterns of 18-year-old Australians:

> Fat intake exceeded 30% of energy in about 80% of subjects and was greater than 40% in about one-quarter. Saturated fat provided more than 10% of dietary energy in more than 90% of participants; less than 1% achieved a polyunsaturated to saturated fat ratio of at least one.
>
> (Milligan *et al.* 1998: 485)

Such information is, of course, translated into a form that lay audiences can understand if it is used as the basis of self-care promotion, but this does not alter the fact that biomedical research necessarily proceeds according to priorities understood in such abstract terms. This has a bearing on the form of self-care advice, as biomedical forms of inquiry tend to produce risk information which is much more useful in the production of individualistic self-care promotion. Professional and institutional authority grants legitimacy to concerns expressed 'from below', and the effect of biomedical dominance over the means of inquiry is that only individualized concerns are legitimated 'from above' by lifestyle health promotion while broader social concerns are largely ignored.

Producing health advice that is empowering to patients relies on the existence of quality research on the meanings of practices and the health priorities of lay people in more concrete terms. Such 'qualitative' research is slowly being accepted in public health but is still framed by the need to collect 'hard data' which is insisted upon within such medically dominated fields (Labonte 1997b).

Reflexivity, modernity and self-consciousness

In order to feel secure, the individual must have faith in experts, in the expert systems they represent and the abstract systems they front. When a popular crisis of faith occurs, experts are wheeled out – the Chairman of the Reserve Bank, the Surgeon General, the Commissioner of Police – to reassure the public and allay fears. The need for public confidence is made problematic, however, by the fact that the form of inquiry on which modern expertise is based relies on critique, scepticism and disagreement. Certainty is dependent upon doubt. In the modern era it was possible to separate the public and private faces of expert systems; in public, the current state of knowledge was proclaimed as indisputable truth, while in private, in research institutions and in boardrooms, the provisional status of current opinion was acknowledged. This front-stage/back-stage separation is becoming increasingly difficult to maintain because intellectual disputes are no longer only of interest to intellectuals. Since lay knowledge is thoroughly infused by and dependent on expertise at so many levels, the potential fallibility of expert knowledge becomes an existential condition for the whole population. It is no longer just science which is founded on shifting sands, as Popper observed – this metaphor now applies to the whole of everyday life (Giddens 1994b: 87). The public is now highly conscious of disputes between experts on a wide range of issues, which has the effect of undermining the authority of any one expert opinion. With the increase in the volume and complexity of expert knowledge production, the stability of the knowledge base decreases and becomes advisory rather than doctrinal (Bauman 1987).

The maintenance of ontological security requires that the individual has a protective cocoon to 'filter out' the more upsetting possibilities and those which are highly improbable, and this filtering process is reliant on trust (Giddens 1991). For example, when driving a car, there are an infinite number of risks which would make concentration impossible were they the constant focus of the driver's attention. The driver is able to feel secure to the extent that they place their trust in others. They trust that other drivers will obey the road laws, trust those who designed, built and maintain the car, trust the engineers who designed the environment in which the car is travelling and the workers who built it. The traffic authorities endeavour to cultivate a degree of insecurity in drivers, however, lest they become too confident on the roads and become careless.

There is a danger here of treating this relationship as the result of a rational evaluation of expert knowledge by lay people. Both Giddens and Beck have often been criticized for their tendency to overemphasize the rational and conscious character of risk perception and lifestyle choices (Petersen 1996). If this were the case, one would expect lay perceptions of the seriousness of a variety of risks to echo expert determinations of their significance, but this appears not to be the case, since there are complex cultural, political and economic forces at work in shaping the lay perception of risks (Gabe 1995; Lidskog 1996). It has long been recognized that simply providing 'objective' information about health risks to the public is usually a very ineffective means of changing self-care behaviour. In the ideal world of those who seek to minimize risk behaviours on a population level, individuals would engage in rational risk calculation when making lifestyle decisions so as to minimize their exposure to risk and maximize their quality of life. As noted above, an early wave of health promotion envisaged that this process would occur quite easily. The task of these early health promotion agencies was to disseminate the latest scientific findings to the public, who would then modify their behaviour accordingly. When this approach failed to yield results, less 'rational' means for the promulgation of risk awareness became the standard tools of those intermediaries who seek to translate particular expert knowledges into lay knowledge in order to change self-care behaviour.

Much health advice employs a superficial understanding of the self, centred on the belief that every aspect of one's self-identity and behaviour is, in principle, open to conscious reflection and modification by a rational actor. This is perhaps most pervasive in self-help literature dealing with the self-management of one's emotional state. By drawing attention to the more superficial dimensions of emotionality and ignoring the deeper and less easily changed characteristics of one's emotional make-up, these texts often contribute to a self-deception which relies on the repression of uncomfortable facts about one's self (Sloan 1987).

Self-care advice must convince its audience that reflexive action can be effective in relation to the particular problem they face. It must first rhetorically 'empower' the reader in relation to their problems, and usually this involves emphasizing the fluidity and mutability of the reader's self-identity, behaviour and circumstances. Within psychotherapeutic self-help literature, for example, there is a nearly unanimous model of emotion which makes overt several assumptions which are necessary conditions for the effectiveness of reflexive 'emotion work'. The dominant model asserts that while emotions are powerful forces in one's life, their causes are not always readily apparent. If emotions are repressed, they re-surface in different forms, and so must be acknowledged as they appear. For a happy and satisfying life, emotions must be made conscious to oneself. Once conscious, they must be worked upon in order to overcome emotional conflict and to reduce negative emotions. Emotional habits and attitudes are learnt, but emotions are also generated in all social intercourse (J. Ryan *et al.* 1994).

Most emotional self-help texts offer cognitive forms of therapy which encourage the reader to introspect and eliminate negative thoughts through rational counter-argument and deliberate positive thinking. This view that one's emotions are open to conscious manipulation is of course much more widespread than self-help books and has also been popular in most forms of personal empowerment psychotherapy such as New Age counsellors and groups, short courses and retreats. The director of Neuro Linguistic Programming's Australian division tells his audience that 'we do have the power of choice. I tell them to do that exercise every day, project those two selves and then reject the depressed self and step into the happy and successful self' (quoted in Freeman 1994: 1). Staying with the example of self-help books, I want to elaborate further this tendency in self-help culture to overstate the ease with which individuals can change their lot – both by ignoring the person's practical conditions of life (solipsism) and by underestimating the ontological depth of the self (cognitivism).

The models of emotions used in self-help literature skirt over the fact that one's emotional make-up is deeply ingrained in one's self-identity, one's worldview, the way one relates to others and the way one cares for one's self. The most fundamental aspects of our emotional lives exist below the level of discursive reflection and provide us with what Giddens (1991) calls a sense of 'basic trust' precisely because they remain unquestioned. Without such an understanding of the depth of emotionality, attempts to change individual patterns of emotionality are bound to be simplistic and ineffective (Wentworth and Ryan 1992). This is, of course, the lesson from psychoanalysis, that the emotional experiences of early childhood are formative of the person's personality but are not readily accessible to the person. We can take from psychoanalysis this depth model, somewhat modified so that the self is conceived in terms of a continuous series of levels of depth which continue to be constituted throughout life rather than the basic structure of personality being fully formed in childhood. Many self-care practices are embedded in the pre-conscious levels of the self through habit in a similar way to the embedding of cultural traditions through repetition of performance (C. Campbell 1996). To take diet, for example, the body becomes accustomed to habitualized practices, and a conscious change to habitual eating practices is likely to cause a bodily reaction, and the same holds for every type of embodied practice. By unrealistically suggesting that by conscious reflection and introspection the person can understand and master every aspect of their own behaviour, emotions and well-being, self-help literature often promotes a naïve voluntarism.

Commercial self-care promotion has an interest in representing the body as a plastic entity that is able to be changed at will. Individuals are persuaded that their bodies are not as fixed and predetermined as they once imagined and that with minimal effort on their part and the purchase of product X they can attain the body they desire rather than having to accept the body they have. The body has become an object of fashion in consumer societies, and the marketing of self-care is reliant on the creation of fashionable diets, fashionable body shapes, fashionable ways to keep fit. In the competition between promoters of self-care practices, there is an inevitable tendency for producers to exaggerate both the benefits of their product and the ease of the behavioural modification being suggested (Rosen 1987). Weight-loss diets are an obvious example of commercial hype being used to sell self-care products and advice which is actually counter-productive, forcing health promotion agencies to spend large amounts of public funds fighting commercial misinformation. Like many behavioural modifications promising instant success, weight-loss diets are unsustainable in the long term, both physiologically and psychologically. Such commercial self-care promotion, in repeatedly and deliberately overstating the individual's capacity to control their own health, individualizes responsibility for health and sits comfortably alongside a neo-liberal concern with handing responsibility back to consumers.

For evidence that the mere provision of information does not change self-care practices significantly, we need not look very far. To take the example of smoking, research on adolescent smoking has found that the two most significant factors in predicting the onset of experimental smoking are peer smoking and depressive symptoms. These factors are important as experimental smokers who have smoked at some point in the past week are twenty-five times more likely than non-smokers to be daily smokers six months on. Given the known relation-ship between nicotine and mood-affecting neuro-transmitters such as seratonin, this finding suggests that the psychological benefits of tobacco use outweigh future health risks especially for those young people who experience depressive symptoms. This is one of the reasons that education raising adolescents' aware-ness of the risks associated with smoking has had little impact on smoking rates amongst young people (Patton 1997). These awareness-raising campaigns operate on a rational model of decision-making which is unable to cope with the deeper psychological determinants of behaviour. The fact of embodiment, of course, constantly places limitations on agency. As biological organisms, humans are programmed with primordial responses which are resistant to conscious attempts to override them (C. Campbell 1996). At an obvious level, the body forces our consciousness to do what it requires – eat, sleep, drink, rest, and so on

– but at another level, the body has desires and predispositions which the conscious actor is often powerless to overcome. As Woody Allen put it, 'the heart wants what the heart wants'.

If it is not difficult to see that psychological depth offers resistance to conscious self-transformation, conversely it is not difficult to show that conscious self-perceptions are easily manipulated by self-help products. In one interesting psychological study, subjects were randomly given a subliminal self-help tape designed either to improve memory or to increase self-esteem. Their self-esteem or memory was tested before and after they had listened to the tape at home over a five-week period. The researchers found that the subliminal self-help tapes did not affect any of the performance measures in a manner consistent with manufacturer claims. However, the subjects' own perceptions of personal improvement were consistent with their expectations. Those who thought they had listened to a self-esteem tape were more likely to believe that their self-esteem had improved and those who thought they had listened to a memory tape were more likely to indicate their memory had improved regardless of the actual subliminal content (Pratkanis *et al.* 1994). Reflexive awareness of the effects of self-help techniques is not a reliable measure of what has happened at deeper levels of consciousness. In many cases, self-help advice may have a placebo effect by increasing the person's perception of control over their condition, which often has positive effects on recovery from illness. Perceived (rather than actual) control over treatment has been consistently related to improved coping in chronic illness (Eitel *et al.* 1995).

Because the distant writer can know very little about the specific situation of the reader, the practical context of the person's conditions of life tends to be largely ignored in self-help literature. Consider, for example, a discussion of stress from an American nursing journal which spells out the steps required for such a dismissal of the conditions of life as a determinant of one's level of stress. It begins by stating that over 95 per cent of all illness and 75 per cent of visits to health-care practitioners are caused by stress. The problem is described. The second stage is to argue that stress is caused not by external events but by the internal psychological processes of the person. The writer argues that 'how an individual views an event determines whether it will be stressful. Nothing is either good or bad, but an individual's perception makes it so' (Wolinski 1993: 721). By connecting the first and second stages of this argument together we have been told that over 95 per cent of all illnesses are caused by problems of individual perception. The third stage is to convince the reader that in order to remedy this situation they should focus more attention on their own inner self and spend less time worrying about the world outside. They should reshape the way they think about things so that they are not so concerned with external affairs. This advice may appeal to a person whose practical context of life presents no great reason for concern but who nonetheless is anxious, and there are surely many people in that category. However, such a dismissal of the practical context undermines any valid concern or resentment held by people whose conditions of life cause them stress. In this way, individualistic self-help advice regularly presents the psychological well-being of the person as existing in a social vacuum. If the world outside of the self is causing pain to a person, they are encouraged to detach themselves from the troubling situation.

In the realm of self-care behaviour, those who seek to change lifestyles, and thereby to instil new self-care knowledges, skills and practices, must first undermine existing practices. This is often achieved by raising anxieties about previously unproblematic behaviour or heightening existing self-doubts. The new beliefs are more consciously adopted than the more habitualized practices which they replace. As a result of these more emotional appeals, postmodern subjects are deliberately reassured and scared many times every day. In order to persuade individuals to act to minimize risks, it is usually necessary to first raise their anxiety about the actual level of risk and the seriousness of the consequences. '*Worry!* – your skin is wrinkling right now! *Don't worry!* – the Ponds Institute have developed a way of preventing wrinkles. *Worry!* – you may live out your old age in poverty! *Don't worry!* – you can secure your future with superannuation.' This perpetual raising and lowering of anxiety produces a subject who has both a high level of anxiety about the future and at the same time is resigned to not being able to do everything possible to minimize all of the risks of which they have been warned. As a result, the islands of certainty and uncertainty which characterize risk consciousness in postmodern societies constitute an ever-changing map of ontological security and anxiety. And this condition is likely to get more intense if, as Bauman says, 'the potential commercial value of risk-fright is infinite' (Bauman 1993: 204).

When faced with an awareness of risk, there are, fundamentally, two responses. One can try to ignore the risk and try to 'live in the present' rather than focusing on a range of possible long-term outcomes. The other alternative is to try to minimize the risk and in doing so remove the source of anxiety. This is not usually a clear-cut choice and such 'decisions' cannot be made on a purely rational basis. The dilemma for self-care promoters is that by adding more information to the pool of risk information which people already possess, they may simply add to the existing information overload, which can as easily lead to fatalism and apathy as to preventive action. Individuals are not only faced with a choice between action and inaction, but are confronted with a range of often conflicting sources of information about the nature of the risk and the efficacy of the courses of action available. As Giddens put it, 'risk calculation has to include the risk of which experts are consulted, or whose authority is to be taken as binding' (Giddens 1994b: 87). In such a world, we seem to be getting further and further from the utopian vision of the health sciences which saw them producing an answer to every health question so that individuals could more live more rationally and be confident in the knowledge that they were doing everything possible to live well.

10 Technological salvation or more human solutions?

- we will never eliminate pain;
- we will not cure all disorders;
- we will certainly die.

Therefore, as sensible creatures, we must face the fact that the pursuit of health may be a sickening disorder. There are no scientific, technological solutions. There is only the daily task of accepting the fragility and contingency of the human situation.

Ivan Illich, Health as one's own responsibility: No, thank you (Illich 1990)

If you watch enough television, you could easily conclude that illness will not going to be troubling human beings for much longer. The cure for every disease seems to lie just around the corner, and if more money was devoted to medical research, the cures would arrive sooner. The mapping of the human genome promises to allow individuals to screen out or head off a huge range of diseases. Public health campaigns aim to stop us dying from smoking, drowning, eating badly, driving too fast or engaging in any behaviour which may damage our health. If all these measures were to be as successful as their publicity makes out, there will soon be nothing left to die of, except, of course, self-neglect. Bauman poetically captures the significance of this 'autonomous strategy', in which responsibility for the implementation of a wide range of new preventive and health-enhancing techniques is put in the hands of activated autonomous individuals:

> At the horizon of the autonomous strategy looms the vision of such a life as may come to an end only through because of the self's neglect of duty, so that the self-contained and self-centred life policy with the care of the body firmly placed at its centre could truly become an adequate and sufficient source of life-meaning. When there are so many means to attend to, who would waste time in examining the ends?
>
> (Bauman 1999: 43)

In this fantasy, the inevitability of death is driven out of awareness so that every effort can be directed towards the project of the self. As I have shown throughout this book, the health-seeking project of the self is now fully integrated into the dominant systems of knowledge production, commodity exchange and mediation of experience. We have seen the amount of health advice in the mass media increase phenomenally in recent decades, as has the extent of expert opinion on the relationship between behaviour and health outcomes, and the proportion of goods and services directed to the care of the self.

These developments have dramatically changed the way people have lived and looked after themselves since the middle of the twentieth century. By the 1960s and early 1970s, when the power of the medical profession was at its peak and social critics were becoming increasingly concerned at the medicalization of everyday life, the medical profession was already beginning to lose its hold over the health beliefs of the population. Alternative sources of health information were providing patients with second opinions even before they stepped into the medical consultation – via magazine articles, radio programmes, government health promotion campaigns and self-help books. This proliferation of information gave rise to a self-help movement determined to empower patients in the face of authoritarian health-care institutions. Passive patients became empowered consumers, at least on a rhetorical level. At the same time, neo-liberal governments became preoccupied with encouraging individuals to take responsibility for themselves as a means of preventing illness and reducing health-care costs. This transformation in the way self-care practices are socially constituted is one important aspect of the radical detraditionalization of the way we live.

Looking to the future, developments in genetic engineering are set to shape health behaviour in the next century in profound ways. On the one hand, advances in genetics could have the effect of reminding us that every person has 'in-built' strengths and susceptibilities which they are powerless to change, thereby shifting the cultural climate away from increasingly obsessive health consciousness to a new form of genetic fatalism. This may prove to be the case in some instances, but what is more likely is that genetic research will actually intensify the perceived need for continual self-discipline in order to maintain one's health. Already genetic screening services are proliferating, offering consumers an increasingly broad-ranging inventory of personal predispositions. The advocates of such techniques of advance warning forcefully point out that such information is intended to empower the person rather than lead to fatalism. The earlier one knows one's susceptibilities, the earlier one can act to improve their future. Thus we are moving into a new phase of the individualization of lifestyle advice in which mail-order genetic screening services compile self-care advice for consumers. In the US, the Great Smokies Diagnostic Laboratory in North Carolina offers 'predictive genomics for personalized medicine' with its Genovations tests, which involve the person sending a vial of used mouthwash to the lab, and two weeks later they receive a tailored programme based on genetic risks (Great Smokies Diagnostic Laboratory 2002). There is obviously huge commercial potential in the genetic individualization of health advice, despite the fact that genetic determinism is already a failing paradigm, since biological causality is distributed at many levels of the human organism and interactions at all these levels are open to numerous environmental, social and behavioural influences (Strohman 2000).

The combined effects of medical, behavioural and biotechnological development will inevitably transform the way we live our lives in the coming decades, but exactly how is anyone's guess. While no one of these technologies is likely to transform everyday life to any great extent, optimistic futurists such as Damien Broderick (1997) foresee a technological convergence in which simultaneous developments in different fields feed into each other to cause seemingly 'magical' social transformations, and a sudden 'spike' in the graph of technological progress. In the history of transportation technology such a 'spike' occurred after the Second World War. The maximum speed at which humans were able to travel had been increasing incrementally for a century but then in just a few years this increased from a couple of hundred kilometres per hour to tens of thousands of kilometres per hour. Broderick predicts such a spike in the development of medical technology between 2030 and 2050 with the cumulative effects of developments in genetic engineering, nanotechnology, cloning and cryogenics.

In the meantime, self-care technophiles are embracing leading-edge biotechnologies, and the most extreme of these seek hi-tech means of overcoming the human condition, usually referring to themselves as transhumanists, posthumanists or extropians. They embrace cosmetic surgery, pharmaceuticals, dietary supplements, artificial body parts, genetic engineering and nanotechnology as ways of improving on the human form, and employ cryogenics as a last resort in the battle to cheat death. The extropians, whom we considered in Chapter 3, understand that to be healthy is to be better than nature intended. To live according to extropian principles one needs money and access to high technology, so it is no surprise that the movement is based in Palo Alto in California's Silicon Valley, where money and science collide. The extropians understand that access to such a 'transhuman' existence is a luxury available only to the few, and consequently are determined to make sure they are part of that privileged minority by placing as much emphasis on financial improvement as they do on physical improvement, supporting radical free-market economics, libertarian social policies and space colonization (More 1994).

Cooperative self-care and political empowerment in self-help groups

In 1935, two chronic alcoholics – one a New York stockbroker and the other an Ohio surgeon – formed the first modern self-help group, Alcoholics Anonymous, and began a movement that has become the principal counter-trend to the dominant form of abstract self-care. Since that time, the number of self-help, or mutual support, groups in the United States and other Western societies has grown exponentially. These groups allow people suffering similar conditions to share experiences and advice through face-to-face interaction, which often leads to organizational structures and political action on behalf of members.

In several important ways, self-help groups represent a counter-trend to the processes that are the focus of this book. Firstly, self-help groups run counter to the trend towards the mediated communication of self-care advice from strangers. Groups are centred on regular face-to-face meetings of people who live near one another, and who attempt to share with and learn from each other as equals with common issues. Secondly, these groups are normally organized by voluntary, not-for-profit associations, which aim to keep costs to a minimum. Health-care providers, pharmaceutical companies and professionals with commercial interests are usually kept deliberately at arm's length from the central concerns of the groups. Thirdly, these groups provide a powerful alternative to rationalized health expertise, by generating knowledge and advice based on lived experience. They enable members to share their experiences within the realm of the meeting room while providing a dynamic means for participants to understand the ways in which the causes and effects of their personal issues are grounded within their society as a whole, and to explore solutions to their private suffering that exist outside of their sphere of individual influence. This capacity of self-help groups to enable individuals to understand their life issues in a broader community context is particularly apparent in groups which seek to utilize collective processes to combat individually experienced stigma and discrimination. I want to explore here the relationships between the therapeutic and political dimensions of the self-help group as a face-to-face means of sharing self-care advice.

Most studies of self-help groups have been carried out by psychologists, psychiatrists and social workers and concentrate on the more therapeutically oriented groups. As a result, most of the available research reflects the more individualistic slant of the self-help groups selected as well as the primary interest of these disciplines in the effectiveness of the group for individual participants (Emerick 1995). A typical approach is that of Levine and Perkins, who have described six general features of self-help groups. They 'promote a psychological sense of community; provide an ideology that serves as a philosophical antidote; provide an opportunity for confession, catharsis and mutual criticism; provide role models; teach effective coping strategies for day-to-day problems; and provide a network of social relationships' (Levine and Perkins 1987: 243). Such a framework, couched in social-psychological terms, reduces the collective project of the group to a series of individual effects, limiting consideration of the social context in which the group operates and in relation to which the group's collective identity is forged. Sadly, there is very little research on the effects of self-help groups on broader cultural and political levels, such as their effects on the popular conceptualization of certain conditions, their effectiveness as advocacy groups or lobby groups.

Between 1935, when Alcoholics Anonymous was formed, and 1975, only a small number of self-help groups existed (Carrol 1994). However, this was to change dramatically. Signs of a shift in attitude were already eveident in the consumer movements that emerged in health care in the late 1960s and early 1970s, whereby patients formed self-help groups in order to cooperate independently of service providers and increase their bargaining power to be able to make demands regarding the quality of care they received (Haug and Lavin 1981). Many popular consumer-oriented texts aimed at empowering patients in relation to their doctors were published in the 1970s, especially in the United States. In 1975 alone the following titles appeared: *How to Choose and Use Your Doctor*(Belsky and Gross 1975); *Talk Back to Your Doctor*(A. Levin 1975); and *How to be Your Own Doctor (Sometimes)*(Schnert 1975). The sentiment of these popular texts is captured in the cover notes from Martin Weitz's *Health Shock* (1982), which warned: 'Routine screening tests, surgery, dentistry, eye care, top-selling drugs including household names – can they do you more harm than good? Many doctors now accept that a large proportion of modern medical treatment is either unnecessary, useless or both.' In 1973, at the beginning of this wave of popular dissent, the American Hospital Association passed the first Patient's Bill of Rights, which was both a set of guidelines for health-care providers and a public relations exercise for hospitals to reassure the public (Schwartz and Biederman 1987: 232). In the intervening decades, this kind of document has become widespread.

Through the flood of mediated health information published in this period, consumers were encouraged to be wary of professional power, to seek out alternative sources of information and to be more self-active in managing their own health rather than passively relying on health-care practitioners, with the result that there was an explosion in the number of self-help groups. In the United States, estimates of the number of self-help groups range between 500,000 and one million, while a Gallup poll in the early 1990s found that 30 per cent of Americans were or had been in a self-help group, and a further 10 per cent were interested but had not got involved (Katz 1993). Other studies estimate that around 60 million Americans have participated in a self-help group at some point in their lives (Davison *et al.* 2000). In Victoria, Australia, the first *Directory of Self-Help Groups*, published by the Council of Self Help Groups in 1981, listed around 150 groups, but within eight years the number of groups listed had grown to 1,000 (Uljar and Hendron 1990). Self-help groups exist outside of the health and disabilities arena (e.g. feminist consciousness-raising groups, residents' associations, etc.), but have been far more dynamic and popular in dealing with questions of identity, embodiment and suffering.

Self-help groups provide a means for people to become active in their own health care, through participation in small groups in which they receive support. In these groups the members' authority as a provider of advice and support rests on their first-hand experience of the condition which brings the group's members together. In this way consumers of health care become (co-)providers of care. Self-help groups generally deal with reactive self-care and usually comprise people (whether we refer to them as patients, clients or sufferers) who are ill or recovering, as well as their families and friends. Those who join self-help groups are often coping with a chronic condition for which they have had little preparation, the experience of which causes them to feel socially and psychologically isolated.

Here I am interested in participatory self-help groups in which the centrality of regular meetings highlights the importance of active participation, rather than 'representative' groups which have a service orientation and in which a small number of members provide services for others. There are, of course, many much older groups oriented to working on behalf of a constituency which can loosely be labelled self-help, such as unions, business groups, lobby groups, consumer groups, and so on. Representative self-help groups differ from the contemporary participatory form under consideration here, however, in that the latter are primarily concerned with personal rather than collective empowerment, with reflexive self-constitution and self-care rather than collective organization and action in the public sphere. Contemporary self-help groups do generally have context-oriented political interests, but, as will be discussed below, these are usually secondary manifestations. Self-help groups serve to establish face-to-face contact and the sharing of experience in a structured forum which is designed to make such face-to-face interaction more efficient. Unlike face-to-face interaction in everyday life, the interaction in self-help groups is compartmentalized as a discrete part of one's life, and is instrumentally oriented to an explicit end. In short, the interaction rarely constitutes a framing level of integration, taking the person out of themselves in a way which extends beyond self-interested therapy.

It is worth distinguishing twelve-step groups, which have adopted the addiction/recovery model pioneered by Alcoholics Anonymous, from non-twelve-step groups. Since the 1960s a range of other twelve-step groups have been started which are directed at changing other types of 'addictive' or compulsive behaviour, including Narcotics Anonymous (1953), Overeaters Anonymous (1965), Gamblers Anonymous (1970) and Co-Dependents Anonymous (1986). The AA model provided a successful formula for the practice of self-help and a philosophical framework which was broad enough to be adaptable to other behavioural problems. By 1992 there were over 130 national twelve-step organizations in the United States, and many more state and local groups (Katz 1993). Central to this philosophical framework of these groups is the twelve-step program developed by AA's founders:

1. We admitted we were powerless over alcohol – that our lives had become unmanageable.

2. Came to believe that a power greater than ourselves could restore us to sanity.

3. Made a decision to turn our will and our lives over to the care of God as we understood Him.

4. Made a searching and fearless moral inventory of ourselves.

5.   Admitted to God, to ourselves, and to another human being the exact nature of our wrongs.

6.   Were entirely ready to have God remove all these defects of character.

7.   Humbly asked Him to remove our shortcomings.

8.   Made a list of persons we had harmed, and became willing to make amends to them all.

9.   Made direct amends to such people wherever possible, except when to do so would injure them or others.

10. Continued to take personal inventory and when we were wrong promptly admitted it.

11. Sought through prayer and meditation to improve our conscious contact with God as we understood Him, praying only for knowledge of His will for us and the power to carry that out.

12. Having had a spiritual awakening as the result of these steps, we tried to carry this message to alcoholics, and to practice these principles in all our affairs.

(cited in Katz 1993: 11–12)

Meetings typically consist of readings, often around one of the steps, followed by participants talking to the groups about significant events, current problems, reflections on the reading, and so on. The twelve-step groups are founded on a premise that behavioural change, at least for those who are addicted, can only be achieved through self-transformation at a spiritual level. The participant must admit powerlessness over their behaviour, an admission that one cannot, by autonomous and conscious efforts, change oneself. Changing one's self, it is argued, requires trust in a higher power, which usually means faith in God, although the degree of Christian spirituality in these groups varies according to the individual group's composition. (On twelve-step self-help groups see Gartner 1985; R. Rogers and McMillin 1989; Kaskutas 1994; Toumbourou and Hamilton 1994.)

The earliest non-twelve-step groups were formed in the late 1940s in the United States by parents of disabled or chronically ill children. The proliferation of local parents' groups soon led to the establishment of national organizations in the early 1950s such as the Association for Retarded Children and the National Haemophilia Foundation (Katz 1993). Some groups are directed at compulsive or addictive behaviour but the majority deal with chronic conditions or rehabilitation, such as Mastectomy Inc. and Mended Hearts in the United

States. Instead of advocating religious transformation through faith in a higher power, they generally focus much more on emotional and psychological dimensions of their shared condition. They are also much more inclined towards the provision of practical advice, coping skills, and so on.

Scientific and medical support for the worth of self-help groups has only been forthcoming, and begrudgingly at that, since epidemiological studies have found that the social support provided by self-help groups tends to increase the body's immunocompetence. There are well-known links between social isolation and poor health practices. Social isolation contributes to depression, undermines one's ability to cope with life stresses, and has been shown to cause physiological changes which increase susceptibility to disease (Berkman and Syme 1979; Petrakis 1988; Katz 1993). Self-help groups have been shown to have measurable effects on the health of participants suffering from serious illness. In 1989, Stanford University psychiatrist David Spiegel's study of breast cancer support groups found that participants lived considerably longer after diagnosis than a control group: thirty-six months compared with nineteen months (Spiegel 1989; Hitch *et al.* 1994). This finding shocked the medical profession, who were prepared to concede that support groups could reduce pain, anxiety and fatigue, but dismissed suggestions of any effect on health on a physiological level. It points to the relationships between social networks, psychological well-being and the functioning of the immune system. In summary, it can be said unequivocally that self-help groups provide personal and social support which improve the health of participants and help them cope with the emotional trauma of illness. (On the therapeutic effects of self-help groups, see R. James 1988; Trojan 1989; Stewart 1990a; Hitch *et al.* 1994.)

People suffering a chronic illness, disability or recovering from stressful or traumatic experiences often feel a sense of isolation, and accompanying social withdrawal, if they believe that no-one around them can understand their condition, and no-one around them can help. Face-to-face interaction between sufferers fosters the realization that there are many other people coping with the same condition. This often has a profound experience on the sufferer, particularly in making sense of the reason for the condition, an issue which can cause much anguish if grappled with in isolation. The realization that the same condition is shared by many others is widely described as a 'consciousness-raising' event, which involves the participants in thinking about broader legal, institutional and cultural impacts on their condition rather than on only a personal level (Levine and Perkins 1987). Friendships often suffer as a result of non-sufferers being unable to come to terms with a sufferer's condition, and so the groups serve as a meeting place for those who will understand them, and who may become important resources in times of crisis (Levine 1988). In most groups, members are encouraged to share distressing experiences and feelings of humiliation, uncertainty and guilt. These are met with sympathetic understanding, forging solidarity based on mutual understanding and shared suffering. Self-help groups aim to create a trusting environment in which criticism and advice are less likely to be received as patronizing or as a threat to one's personal integrity (Levine 1988).

Gartner and Riessman (1977) stress that self-help groups often play a supportive role for people with mental illness. In this model of self-help, the groups provide mutual support networks that may have been lost as part of the experience of living with mental illness. Interestingly, the authors suggest that the self-help groups' support processes provide interpersonal linkages 'that may have been lost or have become disconnected as society has changed' (Gartner and Riessman 1977). While this critical view of societal disconnection reflects a view that community solidarity may have once been 'healthier', it does not, however, automatically lead to a rejection of the socially constructed identities that surround mental illness, especially for many who have experienced the effects of institutionalization.

Professionals tend not to have an extensive knowledge of the day-to-day coping mechanisms routinely employed by sufferers of a particular condition. Because of the isolated occurrence of most of these conditions, sufferers are unlikely to know people in the same condition, and they tend not to write about living with a specific condition. Self-help groups allow for the pooling and trans-mission of practical coping strategies in verbal form (Stewart 1990b). A self-help group participant interviewed in report by the Melbourne-based Health Issues Center captures well the importance of shared experiential knowledge in the following terms: 'When you are in crisis you don't have to explain to them. You don't need to make them understand. When you contact a member of this group there is no need to explain, you get immediate support' (Health Issues Centre 1991: 8). Members of these groups often socialize independently of the group they have met in, and may even provide care for one another on a one-to-one basis. Advocates argue that the popularity of these groups demonstrates that they are meeting a deep need and point to subjective evaluations of participants for evidence of their beneficial effects.

Most self-help groups have a fundamental set of beliefs about the common problem members face. The language of the group often uses terms drawn from the conceptual framework, so that members come to understand their own conditions through the discursive constructions of the group. More experienced members of the groups are often encouraged to take an active part in the group, in many cases becoming group leaders. The presence of people who have over-come the problem that is facing the new member serves as an inspiration, and as concrete evidence of the effectiveness of the group. These people are often fully conversant in the ideology of the group and serve as advocates of its guiding principles (Levine 1988). Many groups, most notably Alcoholics Anonymous and Narcotics Anonymous, stress that it is only through helping others that one's personal coping mechanisms are developed and maintained.

In psychological terms, one of the most fundamental features of the opera-tion of any self-help group is 'cognitive restructuring', which involves changing the way a condition is perceived on a cognitive level, in order that such cognitive changes will alter one's self-concept and behaviour. Thus self-help groups often seek to change the members' and the general population's ideas about the causes of the shared condition (Katz 1993). The sense of empowerment which participants in self-help groups regularly report partly stems from collective discussion and actions geared to changing participants' self-identity and self-care practices (Katz 1993). The positive shared self-image which is thus forged enables one to interact more assertively and confidently with others.

As groups develop over time, many expand their interest to deal also with the more structural causes of the group members' problems. Therapeutic and broader advocacy functions of groups usually exist alongside each other but are emphasized differently by different groups. Frank Riessman, editor-in-chief of *Social Policy*, director of the National Self-Help Clearinghouse and one of the most vocal American advocates of political self-help, observes that groups usually start by 'establishing a shared sense of identity, with the self-help form functioning as a critical step in leveraging them to larger social movement and political action' (Riessman and Bay 1992: 29). He argues that self-help groups inevitably develop a consciousness that 'the personal is political'. Rather than drawing attention away from political issues, in many cases 'the internal identity-strengthening dimension of self-help served as a critical first step that enabled the group to move outward and engage in social and political action' (Riessman and Bay 1992: 34). What we are interested in here is how the introspective components of self-care are framed in such a way that they tie the personal and the political together.

Most self-help groups gradually expand their services over time, shifting from initially being support groups for sufferers to engaging increasingly in more political and educational activities, including advocacy, lobbying, research, and providing information and education to sufferers, professionals and the general public. Most self-help groups publish newsletters with details about group activities, practical information, political and legal issues affecting members, and summaries of new medical research or opinion, and increasingly this publishing is being done on the Web (N. Fox 2001). Larger and more established groups may also provide training classes for health-care workers, establish resource libraries, organize conferences, and even use advertising to attract new members or change public perceptions. While groups maintain their primary therapeutic character for immediate members, the broader services are often carried out on behalf of sufferers generally rather than just the group's participant membership (Health Issues Centre 1991: 12–15). Self-help groups often attempt to redefine and reframe the problems and issues that brought the group together. In coming to terms with their shared condition, the groups often firstly discuss the medical definition of their problem. From that point the condition is often recast as a personal problem, rather than a technical medical one, and later the personal conditions may be related to wider social and political dimensions (Kearney 1991).

Most individual mutual aid groups are affiliated with larger organizations. At the most organized end of the spectrum, Alcoholics Anonymous groups are bound by a shared charter and national and international organizations. Many other groups are organized under the auspices of a broader organization which deals with the demands of sufferers of a particular condition, such as the

Schizophrenia Fellowship. These organizations in turn are often connected with other self-help organizations through 'umbrella' groups, which play a coordinating role in lobbying on behalf of such groups and obtaining the provision of services which individual organizations are unable to muster alone. The Collective of Self-Help Groups (COSHG), the umbrella organization for self-help groups in Victoria, Australia, works towards:

- a more equitable distribution of power and wealth throughout society;
- the furthering of individuals' control over the institutions that affect their lives;
- the development of groups organised by and for people affected by inequalities in society;
- a society free from racism, sexism, ageism, economic exploitation and discrimination based on disability or sexuality.

(cited in Lowther 1997: 6)

In summary, health-related self-help groups can be seen to empower their participants through collective action in three distinct ways. Firstly, they empower patients in relation to their own health through the provision of self-care knowledge, and on an interpersonal level through the creation of a positive self-concept. Secondly, they empower individuals in dealings with health-care practitioners and institutions by having other group members act as patient advocates, and by their increased access to a variety of sources of information about their condition, bureaucratic procedures and their legal rights. Thirdly, they empower the collective membership in relation to the public sphere by changing public perceptions through the mass media, altering policy through lobbying and direct action, engaging in fund-raising to support under-funded services, and so on.

The Right has generally viewed health-related self-help groups as low-cost therapeutic devices. In the United States, the Republican Party platform as early as 1980 called for more self-help initiatives, based on a strong support for the idea of self-reliance and the decreased reliance on state services which this seemed to promise. For decades now, neo-liberal policies have sought to reduce state support to those in need, and replace it with self-help strategies in which sufferers will take more responsibility for their own circumstances. However, in many cases, right-wing governments have proven to be ambivalent towards self-help groups, due to their role in the collective formulation of even stronger demands on the state than had existed before (Lowther 1997: 31).

The Left's interest has been focused on self-help groups as social change agents, emphasizing their capacity for collective action rather than direct therapeutic effects (Riessman and Bay 1992). Such a focus on the politics of the form of self-help groups can be found in the Victorian Council of Self-Help Groups' statement of the 'essential' (read desirable) characteristics of self-help groups, which strongly emphasize the collective power of groups of similarly disenfranchised people:

1   Their membership comprises people who are directly and personally affected by a particular issue, condition or concern. These common concerns or life conditions cause some form of disadvantage or discrimination because rights are denied or specific needs are inadequately met or unfulfilled.

2   They are controlled by members who are directly affected by a particular issue of concern and these members determine what they need and how their needs can best be met.

3   Mutual support is an implicit or explicit function of the group.

(cited in Uljar and Hendron 1990: 8)

For this umbrella organization, it is the act of self-determination by members of their own interests and the democratic and participatory manner in which the scope of the group is determined which is the most important political issue. They see the commonality of the group as centred on a shared experience of disadvantage or discrimination, so their identity is forged through a sense of being outside of, or ignored by, 'society'. The second point addresses empowerment, not in the individualist notion of power over one's self, but as collective self-determination, deciding as a group what the needs of the group are and how to pursue them. The last characteristic distinguishes self-help groups, which have active participants, from service-oriented organizations, which relate to their members only in the manner of consumer participation. According to the Council's principles of self-help, what matters is that a group 'continues to provide mutual support, is controlled by those personally affected by an issue, and demands total accountability from its workers' (cited in Uljar and Hendron 1990: 8).

Tema Okun, a worker in community organizations in the Southern States of America, ponders why the disenfranchised are more interested in self-help than in more overtly political community-level political organizations such as the ones she works in. The answer, in her view, is due to the fact that when people come to progressive political organizations

> they get an impossible work ethic: long hours, low wages, a reinforcement of the race, gender, class and heterosexist power dynamics found outside that doesn't match the rhetoric we speak, and a sense that any attention to personal issues and needs is selfish and wrong.

By contrast, when people become involved in self-help groups,

> they get a place to belong, a place where they are recognized and valued for however they view themselves at the time, a place where others in the group

share their values and validate their experience. They get a place to expose
their fears, get support, feel safe and good about themselves.

(Okun 1992: 45)

The Left, in short, has not paid enough attention to the emotional needs of
those it hopes to attract. Political action has been characterized by the need for
self-sacrifice, and in an era in which the search for self is greater than ever, the
Left has not grasped the fact that the interests of a powerless group include the
emotional well-being of its members, and has been lax in connecting the
personal needs of those people it treats as occupying a structurally determined
position. Okun's advice is that the Left needs to learn more from the lessons of
the women's movement, which was able to bridge the gap between self-oriented
and context-oriented political action.

Reconciling self-care promotion and social support

Self-help groups differ from the other forms of self-care promotion considered in
this book in that they seek to provide tools for self-management within a highly
socialized context, and seek to strengthen the social support available to
members.

As the WHO puts it, social support is '[t]hat assistance available to individuals
and groups from within communities which can provide a buffer against adverse
life events and living conditions, and can provide a positive resource for
enhancing the quality of life' (Nutbeam 1998: 20). Social support comprises
social, emotional and instrumental exchanges which have the effect of making
the person see themselves as an object of value in the eyes of significant others
(Pilisuk and Parks 1986: 17). Such a conception of social support is useful in that
it ties together a number of dimensions of caring relationships. With the erosion
of traditional sources of enduring supportive contact, and the increasing
marginalization of the poor, the experience of loneliness and the feeling of not
being cared for become more widespread (Pilisuk and Parks 1986: 5).

As noted above, the relationship between social support and health is well
known. An increasing number of empirical studies have shown that a lack of
social support is linked to poor health (for example, see Berkman and Syme
1979). This has been especially noted in studies comparing the health of people
in long-term relationships with that of single people, which have repeatedly
shown that the social support received from a partner is a major factor in
ensuring health (Lillard and Waite 1995). There are a number of dimensions to
this relationship between social support and health. As well as providing instrumental support, strong supportive networks assist on an emotional level, firstly by
helping to interpret significant events and hence increasing the person's ability to
cope with stress, and more generally by facilitating a self-perception of being
cared-for, needed and worthy of love (Pilisuk and Parks 1986: 40). Social
marginality, or 'a state of weak and impermanent ties with one's community',
has been shown to have serious detrimental effects on health (Pilisuk and Parks

1986: 32). As well as being caused by poverty and inequality, social marginality can be a short-term disruption, caused by a personal trauma, relocation or some other temporary isolating condition. Extreme cases of long-term marginality are also sometimes caused by physical, mental or intellectual disability, and by the breakdown of significant relationships.

Philip Slater's 1970 book *The Pursuit of Loneliness* was one of the first Left critiques of the new individualism in America, in both its mainstream and counter-cultural manifestations. Slater argued convincingly that the craving for independence and freedom from social constraint is self-defeating. The widespread failure to recognize the fundamental interdependence of people on one another, he argues, has led to a range of existential and cultural anxieties and transferred dependence onto new forms of authority. While the old culture seeks authoritarian and military solutions to social problems, the new culture looks inward with self-transformative and self-enhancing techniques. Because of their individualistic nature, however, Slater argues that these 'efforts at self-enhancement automatically accelerate the very erosion [they seek] to halt' (Slater 1976: 7). Like Lasch and other 1970s critics of cultural narcissism, Slater's point is that individualistic self-help further undermines mutually supportive social ties and therefore the ontological security that comes from being part of a caring community.

Marc Pilisuk and Susan Parks similarly criticize individualistic 'self-indulgence' for eroding social support and hence adding to the health problems of others. 'Each self-indulgent individual', they write, 'removes one potentially committed person from the pool of caring people, leaves one less person upon whom others can invest a sense of trust' (Pilisuk and Parks 1986: 22). Such self-interested behaviour is an abrogation of one's responsibility to others, but it is also self-defeating because every person's physical and mental health relies on them being part of a caring network. Pilisuk and Parks argue that,

> [w]ithout a body of trusted and loved others, our very freedom makes us a slave to whims that cannot be satisfied for want of a standard to know when we have really arrived. [...] With only self-interest as our values, we fall victim to fads, to empty commercial substitutes in a sequence of weekend self-improvement programs.
>
> (Pilisuk and Parks 1986: 22)

By ignoring the social dimension of care, the individual becomes lost in a meaningless and commercial self-help culture that undermines their ontological security by eroding their social connectedness. This is a very important point and one that must be taken into account in any progressive reformulation of self-care. In the next chapter I will sketch out some principles for the production of 'warm' self-care promotion which actually encourages mutual support and which counters the individualistic tendencies described above.

11 Conclusion

Towards a social-ecological approach to self-care promotion

> Few people of attainments take easily to a plan of self-improvement. Some discover very early their perfection cannot endure the insult. Others find their intellectual pleasure lies in the theory, not the practice. Only a few stubborn ones will blunder on, painfully, out of the luxuriant world of their pretensions into the desert of mortification and reward.
>
> Patrick White, *Voss* (1960: 74)

It seems that since Patrick White wrote these words much has changed. Today, many people live with one foot rooted in the habituated practices of everyday life and one foot placed lightly on a myriad of plans for self-improvement. This is especially the case for those 'of attainments', who are over-represented in the ranks of the yoga practitioners, the non-smokers, the health-food consumers and the weekend-retreat goers. In a culture in which all are repeatedly reminded of what they could be doing to improve their health, few people have enough faith in their own perfection that they are insulted at the suggestion that improvement is possible. Many still find their pleasure in the theory of self-improvement rather than the practice, but even they cannot escape the pressure to improve and the burden of responsibility this places on their actions. Today, our pretensions are constantly undermined, leaving us little choice but to wander, with varying degrees of enthusiasm, into that desert of mortification and reward.

In this conclusion I want to draw together the threads of various issues raised throughout this book and synthesize what I see as the positive features of many existing approaches in order to further develop a social-ecological approach to self-care promotion. My objective here is to contribute to the development of progressive responses to the rise of self-care in ways which acknowledge the individualizing tendencies of the detraditionalization of everyday life while avoiding individualistic understandings of contemporary subjectivity. That is, I aim to consider how those committed to egalitarian models of social justice can work through self-care promotion to promote a socially and politically reflexive care of the self. In this conclusion I have not cited examples of the types of approach I am advocating, although similar understandings inform the work of many health promoters, social movement actors, writers and professionals. By this omission I do not mean to ignore those whose work on progressive self-care promotion strategies overlaps with my own. In order to relate the conclusions presented here to the many similar, but more specifically focused, approaches in these fields, continuing work is required, and this is an obvious direction for the further development of the ideas presented in this book. Because the literature in this area is fragmented and scattered across many fields, and because much of it focuses on a specific setting or health issue, drawing the many threads of such thinking together in a coherent way is a formidable, but very important, task for further research on this topic. A central theme of the book has been the nature of the autonomy of the contemporary individual with regard to self-care, and that is where I think we must begin this formulation of a social-ecological approach to self-care promotion.

Autonomy

Just as the legitimacy of the notion of democracy rests on the belief in the autonomy of citizens to choose freely between political options, the legitimacy of the notion of personal responsibility for health rests on the belief in the autonomy of people to choose freely between self-care options. If one acknowledges the orchestrated shaping of the political consciousness of the autonomous citizen by political actors through the increased reach of mass communications, then the regimes we call democratic are more correctly described as 'differentiated and limited autocratic systems', or, in more traditional terms, liberal oligarchies (Zolo 1992). Likewise, in light of the shaping of health consciousness and self-care practices I have outlined in this book, the freedom of the contemporary individual to determine their own health appears illusory, as Rose and others have argued. I have illustrated how, with the dominance of more abstract levels of social integration, the choices exercised over the body are increasingly able to be shaped by corporations, governments, social movements and charismatic individuals. The intensification of self-activating self-care promotion in new approaches to professional practice and through the mass media has allowed for various forms of power to reach more deeply into the shaping of both the reflexive awareness and reflexive practices of the contemporary subject.

If we look at the rise of self-care from the 'bottom up', however, we must acknowledge that this is not how the proliferation of self-care advice is generally experienced. In contemporary Western societies, most people believe (and do not want to be convinced otherwise) that their self-care practices are a dimension of their self-identity which is freely chosen and through which they assert their autonomous individuality. Melucci describes this prevailing sentiment in the following way:

> [O]ur body is the secret place for which we only possess the key of access and where we may return to confirm our experience that we exist as individuals. The body is our unique and unalienable possession which gives us the power of self-recognition in an age when other forms of identification break down
>
> (Melucci 1996: 73)

People seek out reflexive tools to discover themselves in their bodies and to improve their well-being through improving their health. Faced with the often stressful requirement to choose between a plurality of courses of action, people know that their actions are not completely structurally determined. They experience a sense of power over their own lives because they are reminded constantly that it is they who must choose. They receive and seek out conflicting sources of advice from friends, family, colleagues, newspapers, television and professionals. They face the task of sifting through competing claims, conflicting desires, differing risk assessments and an endless number of unwanted anxieties. In this book I have attempted to integrate these two ways of looking at the rise of self-care by theorizing the framing of personal autonomy.

Beyond an emancipatory politics of self-care

Many political responses to the abstraction of self-care seek to heighten the individual's autonomy, liberating the person from constraints that restrict their range of self-care choices. By transcending the power which shapes self-care practices, they argue, the individual can be free to make their own decisions in relation to their health: an anti-institutional politics of self-care aims to liberate the person from the power wielded by the medical profession and health-care institutions; the critics of narcissism dream of an individual able to overcome the pressures of corporate capitalism and the lure of a narcissistic dominant culture in order to be truly inner-directed; and the New Age movement preaches a liberatory self-empowerment which is to be achieved via the introspective scrutinizing and transforming (disembedding) of the socially constructed self, revealing a transcendental 'inner self'. Neo-liberals seek to free the consumer from the constraints imposed by governments and the professions on the market for self-care advice and products. Some feminist writers focus on the structural constraints on women's health choices, arguing that women's choices can only become authentic when the range of options available to them is taken out of the hands of the state and the market and put in the hands of women (Lippman 1999). These all have in common a desire for escape from power that reveals a lack of understanding of the way power operates through the constitution of subjectivity, as well as through restrictions on the field of action. Reducing one's reliance on one form of the constitution of self-care practices increases one's reliance on other forms. These liberatory understandings are appealing as long as attention is focused solely on the power that is being 'transcended' while ignoring the more abstract forms of power that are being entered into. It is often difficult to see how power is exercised through the self-activating forms of self-care promotion, which constitute the individual as free and personally responsible.

In this sense, governmentality theorists are right to point out the illusory nature of the autonomy promoted through the more abstract forms of integration which are becoming dominant in contemporary Western societies. Individualistic self-care promotion often promotes an ideology of autonomy which does not acknowledge the power relations involved in the shaping of the choosing subject. While agreeing with this aspect of Rose's work, we should not follow him in overlooking the ontological conditions in which these activating technologies of power operate. For there is no denying that the contemporary subject is required to exercise more conscious choices over aspects of their 'private' lives which in the past were (comparatively) taken as given. In this sense the *experience* of heightened autonomy is real enough, but is not evenly distributed. The question arising out of this problem, which I believe a progressive politics of self-care must face, is 'how can the power which operates through self-care promotion be made more visible to politically reflexive subjects without trivializing the autonomy which people desire in their private lives?'

A first step is to provide more equal access to the conditions and resources in which meaningful choices are possible. This is increasingly becoming the focus of public health, which seeks to improve the social, economic and environmental preconditions for health, which disproportionately affect the powerless, who are unable to buy their way out of such circumstances. A social-ecological approach of the sort I am advocating would further these efforts by linking the care of the self with the care of others and care for one's social and environmental context. It would present a realistic assessment of the social, physical-environmental, biological and psychological factors that influence one's health and seek to provide practical advice about ways of living that improve the health of the body, mind, society and environment.

One elaboration of such a self-activating politics is Giddens' notion of a 'generative politics' which 'seeks to allow individuals and groups to *make things happen*, rather than have things happen to them, in the context of overall social concerns and goals' (Giddens 1994a: 15). Radical political programmes, he argues, must bring together such a generative politics (which aims at expanding the scope for action) and a life politics (which provides a moral-political framework for the exercise of autonomous action). Generative politics would be facilitated through systems of 'positive welfare', which would be directed to fostering an *autotelic self* in which

> an inner confidence which comes from self-respect, and one where a sense of ontological security, originating in basic trust, allows for the positive appreciation of social difference. It refers to a person able to translate potential threats into rewarding challenges, someone who is able to turn entropy into a consistent flow of experience. The autotelic self does not seek to neutralize risk or to suppose that 'someone will take care of the problem'; risk is confronted as the active challenge which generates self-actualization.
> (Giddens 1994a: 192)

I generally agree with the spirit of Giddens' argument that radical politics must embrace self-active subjectivity rather than continuing to focus simply on the structural constraints on action. If freedom is our fate, we must produce political strategies which work both at an individual level, in helping people to attain the reflexive skills needed to manage their freedom, and at a broader political level, in creating the conditions in which freedoms are more equally distributed. In this conclusion I will seek to elaborate how such a politics could work through social-ecological forms of self-care promotion.

Self-care has been widely seen as a panacea for the ills of institutional care: by governments wanting to shift costs onto the consumers of care; by consumer movements wanting to expand consumer choice; by patients' groups wanting to decrease the power that professionals wield over their lives. While in many cases the motivation behind such calls is laudable, very often the informational and material resources needed for self-care are not taken into account, as was the case with the intellectual expression of this sentiment by critics of medicalization such as Illich and Zola, who failed to see that the constitution of self-care practices was taking place increasingly through the mass media and was increasingly commercialized.

Community-based services which use the self-care capacity of individuals have been widely implemented as alternatives to institutional care in hospitals (through early-discharge policies), nursing homes and psychiatric hospitals as cost-saving or, more accurately, cost-shifting measures. In such cases, self-care models have the potential to foster independent living and decision-making, but such autonomy is dependent on the provision of coordinated information, care and services by various health and social service professionals (for an example of such an approach, see Cates 1993). Generally, such de-institutionalization has been successful when the needs of patients have been provided for in novel ways as part of this process, but in many cases simple cost-cutting measures have used the language of patient empowerment without providing the resources needed. The most striking example of this is the dramatic increase in the numbers of homeless mentally ill people in the United States as a result of the de-institutionalization of mental health care.

De-institutionalization does not of itself result in greater independence; instead it results in greater dependence on face-to-face care provided within the family, on disembodied sources of self-care advice and on limited access to professional care. In this area, individualistic understandings of self-care have legitimated policies which have left many vulnerable people feeling abandoned by health-care systems.

Contextualizing self-awareness

One of the major political problems with individualistic approaches to self-care promotion is the atomistic and superficial self-awareness they encourage. Self-care practices are seen as freely chosen in a social vacuum by conscious actors, causing the recipients of such advice to look inside themselves for both explanations and solutions. If they reflect on broader issues or deeper levels of subjectivity, it is to explain the causes of existing patterns of self-care, but most often the solutions posed involve only the conscious action of the individual. The message is conveyed that 'even if you are not directly responsible for the problem, you are responsible for the solution'. A social-ecological approach would encourage a broader form of self-awareness, incorporating both a 'deeper' and more complex understanding of subjectivity and a more developed account of the social shaping of reflexive behaviour.

With regard to the first of these, social-ecological self-care promotion would encourage an understanding that there is a depth to the psyche which is not easily able to be reflected upon or changed. This involves accepting that there are deep psychological limitations on reflexive action and 'cognitive restructuring'. For example, when dealing with those who are depressed and who have a family history of depression, it is irresponsible to suggest that they can by acts of will transform their basic outlook into that of a cheerful optimist. For the psychologically trained, of course, such comments are so obvious and rudimentary as to not need stating. I am aware that any brief discussion of psychological resistance to self-transformation entered into here is only able to touch on these issues, but this is a point worth making given the extent of simplistic and voluntaristic understandings in popular self-help advice. Regardless of whether such deep structures of the personality are held to be of social or biological origin, it should be acknowledged that these aspects of the person's make-up will continue to exert an influence. Self-care promotion can encourage the person to be more aware of the deeper elements of their psyche and to develop strategies to draw on those fundamental aspects of their personality they like and to allow them to deal with those aspects of themselves which they do not like but cannot change. The message is that certain psychological features of the person that shape their desires and anxieties, and thus their self-care practices, can only be understood, not transformed.

Self-care practices are usually habitualized and pre-conscious. They are usually able to be made more conscious by reflection on one's own behaviour and worked upon, but this does not mean that they can be so easily 'reinscribed'. There is an intractability to routinized self-care practices which self-care promotion has a responsibility to be honest about, despite the temptation to try to boost the person's motivation by promising quick success in self-transformation. The patterns in one's self-care practices can be made visible, but the reasons for the intractability of such practices are often more difficult to discover. Take a simple example like drinking too much coffee. A person may become aware of the health consequences of drinking too much coffee, reflect on their own coffee-drinking habits, count the number of cups they drink each day, and then decide that they drink too much. The desire for coffee persists, however. Further reflection is required to understand the nature of the desire for coffee, and if the desire is persistent and strong enough, this could lead the person into deeper and deeper introspection without ever yielding an explanation capable of being translated into effective self-transformative techniques. It is important to bear in mind that the inner self is deeply constituted through social relationships on many levels, and in emphasizing the social relations of self-care there is no clear distinction between self and society. Contextual approaches to self-care promotion encourage an understanding of the self as socially constituted in an ongoing manner, and seek to link the psychological processes which underlie self-care with the social relations in which they are constituted. In this sense, developing self-awareness involves developing an awareness of the way one's own beliefs and practices are shaped through social relations of various types. Below I will address the social and ecological contextualization of self-care in more detail, but I want firstly to discuss how such a contextual approach could deal with issues of social inequality.

Tackling social inequality through self-care promotion

As many on the Left have pointed out, self-care promotion presents two major problems for those who seek to reduce social inequality. Firstly, much self-care promotion is victim-blaming. By emphasizing the capacity of the individual actively to determine their health status, self-care promotion very often under-emphasizes or completely ignores the social, psychological and biological conditions which shape individual behaviour, thus implying that the individual alone is responsible for health outcomes. Those whose self-care practices result in poor health (more often the powerless and the poor) are held personally responsible, directing political attention away from the social conditions which influence one's health and which shape self-care practices. Secondly, self-care promotion is more effective in changing the behaviour of the already healthier sections of society – the educated and the wealthy. By improving the health status of the middle class more than the working class, and the healthy more than the chronically ill, self-care promotion has had a regressive effect by widening inequalities in health status.

So, for good reason, the Left is generally highly suspicious of self-care promotion approaches to improving public health and has instead concentrated on the material foundations for health. While I do not in any way want to be critical of the work of public health associations to redress the iniquitous distribution of socially produced health risks, by refusing to participate in self-care promotion the Left leaves the shaping of the health beliefs and self-care practices of the population to more conservative political forces and the market, who have few qualms about the social inequalities which individualistic self-care promotion perpetuates. A more thoroughly theorized contextual approach to self-care promotion, I believe, would allow those on the Left to become more wholeheartedly and constructively engaged in self-care promotion. So how could a contextual self-care promotion redress the inequalities in health rather than exacerbating them, as individualistic and commercial self-care promotion has tended to do?

Progressive self-care promotion works alongside and is coordinated with settings approaches which tackle underlying social factors. Self-care advice and information should not be afraid to point to the unequal access to the resources required for self-care and should seek to increase a political reflexivity as to the social and political causes of the unequal distribution of health risks. For example, in relation to smoking and illicit drug use, the reasons why the poor use cigarettes and other drugs more should be openly discussed. In this way anti-smoking campaigns and harm-reduction strategies for illicit drug use could seek to make their audiences more aware of the ways in which the experience of poverty encourages such potentially self-destructive but pleasurable practices. Such effects of social disadvantage might include: the stress produced by poor working conditions; the anxiety produced by the financial precariousness of those at the bottom end of deregulated, 'flexible' labour markets; the despair of those young people who can see no way of overcoming their social disadvantage; the loss of self-esteem which comes with poverty in societies in which wealth is associated with personal success; the prospect of living out one's old age in poverty, which makes 'premature' death seem less foreboding; and the reduced availability of 'healthier' but more expensive forms of stress relief, relaxation and embodied pleasure which are used by the wealthy. Such a political slant would focus attention on the effects of deprivation, encouraging action on the causes of social inequality rather than blaming its victims. Those who recognize their own experiences described in the course of such self-care promotion may still continue to engage in potentially self-destructive behaviours, but such an under-standing of the social contexts of their actions is, I believe, more likely to improve the person's self-esteem and therefore subjective well-being rather than reinforcing self-blame and feelings of personal inadequacy. Such a contextual self-care promotion would encourage more 'self-constructive', rather than self-destructive, ways of dealing with such conditions through individual, collective and political measures.

Such an approach seeks to make audiences aware of the conditions which frame personal autonomy, reminding the public that the choices available and the attractiveness of those options are profoundly shaped by social and economic factors. This does not downplay the autonomy of the person but seeks to help the person to reflect on the material and psychological conditions under which their autonomy is exercised. Such an approach is in line with Bauman's argu-ment that contemporary political strategies should respond to the individualistic desire for personal freedom with a 'reassertion of the right of free individuals to secure and perpetuate the conditions of their freedom' (Bauman 1997: 207). Because of this focus on the conditions of freedom, contextual self-care promo-tion is designed to be more useful to those who need it most. To stay with the present example, consider those who use cigarettes and illicit drugs but whose conditions of life do not expose them to pressures of the same magnitude. In this group, an understanding of the social contexts which partially explain such prac-tices would be of benefit in developing a sense of compassion for the poor, and would at the same time lead them to see their own behaviour as relatively more freely chosen. If there is to be a burden of responsibility for the consequences of such actions, those who are better-off are seen to be more freely responsible for the choices they make, which inverts the tendency of individualistic self-care to blame the poor, who engage in such self-destructive practices in greater numbers.

Reflexivity in the production of self-care promotion

For social-ecological self-care promotion to be effective, those engaged in self-care promotion would need to maintain a reflexive awareness of their own capacities and limitations by understanding its relationship to the dominant modes of practice which frame the production of self-care in contemporary societies. As I discussed in Chapter 4, popular practices of self-care have been transformed by the dominance of the commodity form of production, the mass media and technoscientific inquiry, and, in order to avoid replicating the individualistic forms of self-care promotion which these dominant modes of practice have tended to encourage, contextual self-care promoters must be aware of their place within this broader constellation. At this point I merely want to revisit some of the issues which self-care producers cannot escape, in order to provide an indication of the type of reflexivity I am proposing.

For those working in the private sector, this means being aware of the logic of the market which frames the conditions of possibility for their work. Commercial self-care promotion is, of course, primarily motivated by the profits which are available to those who can effectively tap into the anxieties and desires of potential consumers. As a result, these forms of self-care promotion tend to take advantage of health concerns indiscriminately, strategically heightening or promising reassurance of those concerns which prove beneficial to the producer. This is a structural feature of the contemporary market which all commodified self-care advice, information and products must work within. The publishing industry provided an example of the way in which competition between producers (writers and publishers) has led to the production of high-turnover, short shelf-life self-help books and magazines which have a commercial incentive to make extravagant claims and promise simplistic solutions to complex problems. Weight-loss dietary fads are one expression of this tendency. For decades, magazine publishers have been exploiting women's anxieties over body image by filling their publications with a succession of short-term solutions which encourage women to try diet after diet, even though this form of dieting is known to be counterproductive as far as weight loss is concerned. The pages in these magazines alternate dietary and other self-care advice with fashion shoots and advertisements which fuel the desire for desire for a thinner body and heighten dissatisfaction with one's present body image. In order to counter such exploitation, self-care promoters working in the private sector must be constantly vigilant against commercial pressures which threaten to undermine any political or public health concerns if they prove less profitable. Those working in the public sector, for non-profit organizations or in political organizations must be aware that the self-care promotion they produce is also framed by the dominance of the commodity form, reaching a public which is already inundated with commercial self-care messages. Whether in the private or public sectors, the work of self-care promoters takes the form of a commodified labour relation in which they sell their intellectual labour to an employer, and, like private employers, the state has its own interests to serve, such as using self-care to justify cuts to services or emphasizing personal responsibility to divert political pressure away from social causes of illness.

Self-care promoters must also be aware of the power and limitations of the means of communication through which self-care advice is disseminated. Compared with mediated advice, the clinical setting allows health-care professionals to have a more reciprocal relationship with those who are consulting them, within time/money constraints. Working through the mass media provides the self-care promoter with very little knowledge of the specific social contexts of their audience. This can be overcome to some extent by more closely targeted communications aimed at a specific audience and by producers having a good understanding of their audience through other forms of interaction. Nevertheless, mediated self-care promotion is necessarily much more generic than face-to-face interaction, and its reception is inherently unpredictable. I will discuss these issues in more detail in the section below.

The third dimension of the reflexive awareness of the framing of self-care promoters is in relation to the technoscientific mode of inquiry. Self-care promoters need to understand how the form of intellectual inquiry affects the form of the information at their disposal. With the dominance in public health of statistically based epidemiological approaches, a considerable amount of knowledge about abstract health risks is produced. The form which this knowledge takes is oriented towards biomedical disease-prevention models. In this type of inquiry, self-care practices are broken up into discrete components to reduce ways of living to quantifiable data suitable for the research methodologies being used. Similarly, states of health and illness are broken down into narrowly defined biomedical categories. As a result, correlations are determined between specific behavioural practices and specific disease states. This information is fed back to self-care promoters, who often have little choice at this stage other than to work within such narrow and individualistic understandings of the relationships between ways of life and health. This presents a major challenge for contextual approaches to self-care promotion; biomedical research findings generally have very little significance once health-related behaviours are viewed in the context of the social relations in which they are practised and constituted. At the same time, the health concerns which are identified by such research may have very little meaning for lay people, who understand their health in more general terms rather than as a list of probabilities of incurring various diseases. In order to avoid the individualization of risk management which results from the proliferation of such decontextualized health information, contextual self-care promotion must draw on forms of inquiry which study self-care as socially constituted and socially meaningful practices. This research should as far as possible be directed by the health priorities of those to whom it is intended to be of benefit. To return to the example of poverty and drug use, I would suggest that the type of research that this group would find most useful in improving their well-being would be highly incompatible with the dominant modes of inquiry. Likewise, the implicit notion of health which would guide the self-care practices of this group would be very different from that which underlies biomedical research. It is important that contextual self-care promoters be aware of the ways in which various forms of inquiry impact upon their practice, and they must seek to change research priorities to ensure the production of knowledge appropriate to the socially defined ends they are working towards.

Promoting self-care across levels of integration

Much of the argument of this book centres on the need to develop self-care promotion which engages with the integration of the person across different levels of abstraction. With the intensification of more abstract forms of the constitution of self-care practices, the significance of ongoing face-to-face relationships has too often been overlooked and undermined. A crucial task for social-ecological self-care promotion is to encourage close, mutually rewarding supportive relationships in which people care for each other and provide self-care resources and advice in less structured but deeply connected ways.

When operating through professional consultation or the media, this means producing 'warm' advice which encourages individuals to build and maintain lasting mutually supportive relationships, sharing their own knowledge and drawing on the first-hand experience of others. In this way, self-care promotion can seek to counter the many forces which militate against such social support by cultivating an understanding that the sense of self-worth which comes from being cared about and cared for by others plays an important role in shaping the care of the self. In detraditionalized societies, increasingly socially isolated individuals need to be more actively supported by those around them in order to deal with the precariousness both of contemporary relationships and of the conditions of life. The freedom of the contemporary subject places strains on ontological security, which requires active shoring up in the context of trusting relationships with significant others.

At the professional-institutional level, a more contextual approach would see self-care promoters working with specific communities and in specific social settings in order to set priorities and develop strategies which are arrived at through participatory means and which are most useful to the people whom they are intended to assist (Labonte 1997a). In both community-based health promotion and clinical practice, professionals should seek to integrate informal ongoing social support with self-help groups and appropriate mediated sources of information such as videos, audiotapes, books and information sheets. In producing such mediated self-care promotion techniques, a contextual approach would use the specific medium in ways which enhance rather than undermine these less abstract relationships. A contextual approach would encourage the person to evaluate the suitability of the advice being provided in light of their own experience and discuss the issues with significant others and health-care professionals. Such forms of self-care promotion should draw the person's attention towards social contexts which shape their self-care practices, warning them to be wary of quick-fix solutions, superficial explanations and unsustainable short-term behavioural modification plans. In summary, such abstract forms of self-care promotion can be used in ways which enhance and encourage more concrete relationships with both professionals and lay people, encouraging their audience to work to establish relationships of mutual understanding with professionals they can relate to and who can provide the support and advice they require, and, at the same time, emphasizing the importance of caring relationships wherever they may be found.

Bibliography

Ackroyd, A. (1997) 'Have I got a life for you', *The Age* (Melbourne) 13 September: 24–6.

Albanese, C. (1990) *Nature Religion in America*, London: University of Chicago Press.

Alder, V.S. (1968) *The Finding of the Third Eye*, London: Rider.

Alonzo, A. (1993) 'Health behaviour: issues, contradictions and dilemmas', *Social Science and Medicine* 37, 8: 1019–34.

Althusser, L. (1969) *For Marx*, Harmondsworth: Penguin.

___ (1977) *Lenin and Philosophy*, New York: Monthly Review Press.

American Academy of Pediatrics (1999) 'Media education', *Pediatrics* 104, 2: 341–3.

Anti-Cancer Council of Victoria (1990) *Tobacco Action Pack 7: Tobacco Advertising and Sponsorship*, Carlton South: Anti-Cancer Council of Victoria.

Apodimi Compania (1992) *Melisma*, Audio Compact Disc, Melbourne: Brunswick Recordings.

Armstrong, D. (1983) *Political Anatomy of the Body: Medical Knowledge in Britain in the Twentieth Century*, Cambridge: Cambridge University Press.

___ (1984) 'The patient's view', *Social Science and Medicine* 18, 9: 737–44.

___ (1985) 'The subject and the social in medicine: an appreciation of Michel Foucault', *Sociology of Health and Illness* 7, 1: 108–17.

___ (1988) 'Historical origins of health behaviour', in R. Anderson, J. Davies, I. Kickbusch, D. McQueen and J. Turner (eds) *Health Behaviour Research and Health Promotion*, Oxford: Oxford University Press.

Australian Medical Association (1997) *Media Release: Shock Tactics Work in Selling Health Messages*, Melbourne: Australian Medical Association.

Bachu, A. and O'Connell, M. (2001) *Fertility of American Women June 2000: Population Characteristics*, Washington, DC: US Census Bureau. Online Available HTTP *http://www.census.gov/prod/2001pubs/p20–543rv.pdf*

Bauman, Z. (1987) *Legislators and Interpreters: On Modernity, Post-modernity and Intellectuals*, Cambridge: Polity Press.

___ (1988) *Freedom*, Milton Keynes: Open University Press.

___ (1993) *Postmodern Ethics*, Oxford: Blackwell.

___ (1997) *Postmodernity and its Discontents*, Cambridge: Polity Press.

___ (1999) *In Search of Politics*, Cambridge: Polity Press.

Beattie, A. (1991) 'Knowledge and control in health promotion: a test case for social policy and social theory', in J. Gabe, M. Calnan and M. Bury (eds) *The Sociology of the Health Service*, London and New York: Routledge.

Beck, U. (1992) *Risk Society: Towards a New Modernity*, London: Sage.

___ (1994) 'The reinvention of politics: towards a theory of reflexive modernization', in U. Beck, A. Giddens and S. Lash (eds) *Reflexive Modernization: Politics, Tradition and Aesthetics in the Modern Social Order*, Cambridge: Cambridge: Polity Press.

Beck, U. and Beck-Gernsheim, E. (1996) 'Individuation and "precarious freedoms": perspectives and controversies of a subject-oriented sociology', in P. Heelas, S. Lash and P. Morris (eds) *Detraditionalization: Critical Reflections on Authority and Identity, Oxford and Cambridge, MA*: Blackwell.

Becker, M. (1974) 'The health belief model and personal health behavior', *Health Education Monographs* 2: 326–473.

Bell, D. (1976) *The Cultural Contradictions of Capitalism*, London: Heinemann.

Bellah, R., Madsen, R., Sullivan, W.M., Swidler, A. and Topton, S.M. (1985) *Habits of the Heart: Individualism and Commitment in American Life*, Berkeley: University of California Press.

Belsky, M. and Gross, L. (1975) *How to Choose and Use Your Doctor: the Smart Patient's Way to a Longer, Healthier Life*, New York: Arbor House.

Bennett, W. (1996) *The best welfare reform: end it.* Empower America. Online Available HTTP *http://townhall.com/empower/welfare-bestref.html*

Bennett, W. and Wehner, P. (1996) *Competing themes in the welfare debate.* Empower America. Online Available HTTP *http://townhall.com/empower/welfare-compete.html*

Berkman, L. and Syme, L. (1979) 'Social networks, host resistance and mortality: a nine-year follow-up study of Alameda County residents', *American Journal of Epidemiology* 109, 2: 186–204.

Berman, M. (1982) *All That is Solid Melts into Air: the Experience of Modernity*, New York: Simon and Schuster.

Bessant, J. (1994) 'Feral policy: the politics of the "underclass" debate', *Arena Magazine* 10: 23–4.

Better Health Commission (1986) *Looking Forward to Better Health*, Canberra: Australian Government Printing Service.

Blake, J. (1977) 'From Buchan to Fishbein: the literature of domestic medicine', in G. Risse, R. Numbers and J.W. Leavitt (eds) *Medicine without Doctors: Home Healthcare in American History*, New York: Science History Publications.

Bouhoutsos, J., Goodchilds, J. and Huddy, L. (1986) 'Media psychology: an empirical study of radio call-in programs', *Professional Psychology: Research and Practice* 17, 5: 408–14.

Bourdieu, P. (1978) 'Sport and social class', *Social Science Information* 17, 6: 819–40.

___ (1990) *The Logic of Practice*, Cambridge: Polity Press.

___ (1993) 'How can one be a sports fan?' in S. During (ed.) *The Cultural Studies Reader*, London and New York: Routledge.

British Medical Association (1993) *Complementary Medicine: New Approaches to Good Practice*, Oxford: Oxford University Press.

Brittan, A. (1977) *The Privatised World*, London: Routledge and Kegan Paul.

Broderick, D. (1997) *The Spike: Accelerating into an Unimaginable Future*, Kew: Reed.

Brodie, M., Foehr, U., Rideout, V., Baer, N., Miller, C., Flournoy, R. and Altman, D. (2001) 'Communicating health information through the entertainment media', *Health Affairs* 20, 1: 192–9.

Brow, J. (1997) 'Bare facts better than shock tactics, health survey finds', *The Age* (Melbourne) 23 July.

Brown, P.A. and Piper, S.M. (1995) 'Empowerment or social control? Differing interpreta-tions of psychology in health education', *Health Education Journal* 54: 115–23.

Brown, S. and Szoke, H. (1988) 'Health promotion: the Victorian context', *Health Issues* 14: 35–9.

Burchell, G. (1996) 'Liberal government and techniques of the self', in A. Barry, T. Osborne and N. Rose (eds) *Foucault and Political Reason: Liberalism, Neo-Liberalism and Rationalities of Government*, London: University College London Press.

Campbell, C. (1996) 'Detraditionalization, character and the limits to agency', in P. Heelas, S. Lash and P. Morris (eds) *Detraditionalization: Critical Reflections on Authority and Identity*, Oxford and Cambridge, MA: Blackwell.

Campbell, R. (1995) 'Smoking becomes a rights issue as company cashes in', *Canberra Times* 30 April: 1.

Cancian, F. and Gordon, S. (1988) 'Changing emotion norms: love and anger in US women's magazines since 1900', *Gender and Society* 2: 308–42.

Carnegie, D. (1962) *How to Stop Worrying and Start Living*, Kingswood: Cedar Books.

Carrol, D. (1994) 'Self-help and the new health agenda', *Social Policy* Spring: 44–52.

Castel, R. (1991) 'From dangerousness to risk', in G. Burchell, C. Gordon and P. Miller (eds) *The Foucault Effect: Studies in Governmentality*, Hemel Hempstead: Harvester Wheat-sheaf.

Cates, N. (1993) 'Trends in care and services for elderly individuals in Denmark and Sweden', *International Journal of Aging & Human Development* 37, 4: 271–6.

Clarfield, M. (1997) 'Self-help medical advice was popular in the 1930s, too', *Canadian Medical Association Journal* 157, 9: 1272–3.

Coffey-Lewis, L. (1982) *Be Restored to Health: How to Manage Stress, Heal Your Self and Be Whole Again*, Toronto: Personal Library.

Collier, J.L. (1991) *The Rise of Selfishness in America*, New York: Oxford University Press.

Connolly, W. (1992) 'Discipline, politics, ambiguity', in T. Strong (ed.) *The Self and the Polit-ical Order*, Oxford: Blackwell.

Conrad, P. (1994) 'Wellness as virtue: morality and the pursuit of health', *Culture, Medicine and Psychiatry* 18: 385–401.

Coonan, W., Worsley, A. and Maynard, E. (1986) *Body Owner's Manual for Secondary Students and Their Parents*, Adelaide: Education Department of South Australia Publications Branch.

Cooper, P.J., Coker, S. and Fleming, C. (1994) 'Self-help for bulimia nervosa – a prelimi-nary report', *International Journal of Eating Disorders* 16, 4: 401–4.

Coreil, J. and Levin, J. (1984) 'A critique of the life style concept in public health educa-tion', *International Quarterly of Community Health Education* 5, 2: 103–14.

Coreil, J., Levin, J. and Jaco, E.G. (1985) 'Life style- an emergent concept in the sociomedical sciences', *Culture, Medicine and Psychiatry* 9: 423–37.

Coward, R. (1989) *The Whole Truth: the Myth of Alternative Health*, London: Faber.

Cowley, G. (2002) 'Now, "Integrative" Care', *Newsweek* 2 December: 46–53.

Crawford, R. (1977) 'You are dangerous to your health: the ideology of victim blaming', *International Journal of Health Services* 7: 663–80.

—— (1979) 'Individual responsibility and health politics in the 1970s', in S. Reverby and D. Rosner (eds) *Health Care in America*, Philadelphia: Temple University Press.

—— (1980) 'Healthism and the medicalization of everyday life', *International Journal of Health Services* 10: 365–88.

Crossley, N. (1996) 'Body-subject/body-power: agency, inscription and control in Foucault and Merleau-Ponty', *Body and Society* 2, 2: 99–116.

Davidson, L., Chapman, S. and Hull, C. (1979) *Health Promotion in Australia*, Canberra: Australian Government Printing Service.

Davis, R. and Miller, L. (1999) 'Millions comb the Web for medical info', *USA Today* 15 August.

Davison, K.P., Pennebaker, J.W. and Dickerson, S.S. (2000) 'Who talks? The social psychology of illness support groups', *American Psychologist* 55: 205–17.

Davy, J. (1994) *Health Moves: Senior Personal Development, Health and Physical Education*, Port Melbourne: Rigby Heinemann.

Dean, K. (1986) 'Lay care in illness', *Social Science and Medicine* 22: 275–84.

DeFriese, G. and Woomert, A. (1982) 'The policy implications of self-care in the study of health and illness behaviour', *Social Policy* Fall: 55–8.

Denfeld, R. (1995) *The New Victorians: a Young Woman's Challenge to the Old Feminist Order*, St Leonards: Allen and Unwin.

Department of Health and Social Security (1976) *Prevention and Health: Everybody's Business*, London: Her Majesty's Stationery Office.

Diamond, H. and Diamond, M. (1986) *Fit For Life: the Natural Body Cycle, Permanent Weight-Loss Plan That Proves It's Not What You Eat, But When and How!*, North Ryde: Angus and Robertson.

Dill, A., Brown, P., Ciambrone, D. and Rakowski, W. (1995) 'The meaning and practice of self-care by older adults: a qualitative assessment', *Research on Aging* 17, 1: 8–41.

Dixon-Woods, M. (2001) 'Writing wrongs? An analysis of published discourses about the use of patient information leaflets', *Social Science and Medicine* 52: 1417–32.

Dubos, R. (1960) *Mirage of Health*, London: Allen and Unwin.

—— (1968) *Man, Medicine and Environment*, London: Pall Mall Press.

Duckett, S. (1997) 'Tobacco control in Victoria', *Health Promotion Matters*, 1 May: 4–5.

Easthope, G. (1993) 'The response of orthodox medicine to the challenge of alternative medicine in Australia', *Australian and New Zealand Journal of Sociology* 29, 3: 289–301.

Eaton, S.B., Shostak, M. and Konner, M. (1988) *The Paleolithic Prescription: a Program of Diet and Exercise and a Design for Living*, New York: Harper and Row.

Ehrenreich, B. (1989) *Fear of Falling: the Inner Life of the Middle Class*, New York: Pantheon Books.

Ehrenreich, J. (1978) 'Introduction: the cultural crisis of modern medicine', in J. Ehrenreich (ed.) *The Cultural Crisis of Modern Medicine*, New York: Monthly Review Press.

Eisenberg, D., Kessler, R., Foster, C., Norlock, F., Calkins, D. and Delbanco, T. (1993) 'Unconventional medicine in the United States: prevalence, costs and patterns of use', *The New England Journal of Medicine* 328, 4: 246–52.

Eitel, P., Hatchett, L., Friend, R., Griffin, K.W. and Wadhwa, N.K. (1995) 'Burden of self-care in seriously ill patients – impact on adjustment', *Health Psychology* 14, 5: 457–63.

Elias, N. (1978) *The Civilizing Process: Volume One — The History of Manners*, Oxford: Blackwell.

—— (1991a) 'Individualization and the social process', in M. Schröter (ed.) *Norbert Elias: the Society of Individuals*, Oxford: Blackwell.

—— (1991b) 'Wishful and fear-inspired self-images of human beings as individuals and society', in M. Schröter (ed.) *Norbert Elias: the Society of Individuals*, Oxford: Blackwell.

Emerick, R. (1995) 'Clients as claims makers in the self-help movement: individual and social change ideologies in former mental patient self-help newsletters', *Psychosocial Rehabilitation Journal* 18, 3: 17–35.

Empower America (1996) *Principles for real welfare reform.* Empower America. Online Available HTTP *http://townhall.com/empower/welfare-ibwelfare.html*

Engels, F. (1973) *The Condition of the Working Class in England: From Personal Observation and Authentic Sources,* Moscow: Progress Publishers.

Ernst, E. (1994) 'Complementary medicine: changing attitudes', *Complementary Therapies in Medicine* 2: 121–2.

European Commission (2002) *Commission Recommends Quality Criteria for Health Websites.* Brussels: European Commission. Online Available HTTP *http://europa.eu.int/information_society/eeurope/ehealth/index_en.html* (24 January 2003).

Featherstone, M. (1987) 'Lifestyle and consumer culture', *Theory, Culture and Society* 4: 55–70.

___ (1991) *The Body: Social Process and Cultural Theory,* London: Sage.

Finerman, R. and Bennett, L. (1995) 'Guilt, blame and shame in sickness', *Social Science and Medicine* 40, 1: 1–3.

Fisher, S. (1991) 'A discourse of the social: medical talk/power talk/oppositional talk', *Discourse and Society* 2, 2: 157–82.

Flora, J. and Wallack, L. (1990) 'Health promotion and mass media use: translating research into practice', *Health Education Research: Theory and Practice* 5, 1: 73–80.

Foucault, M. (1965) *Madness and Civilization: a History of Insanity in the Age of Reason,* New York: Pantheon.

___ (1977) *Discipline and Punish: the Birth of the Prison,* Harmondsworth: Penguin.

___ (1980) 'Two lectures', in C. Gordon (ed.) *Michel Foucault: Power/Knowledge,* New York: Pantheon.

___ (1981) *The History of Sexuality,* Harmondsworth: Penguin.

___ (1982) 'The subject and power', *Critical Inquiry* 8: 777–95.

___ (1988) 'Technologies of the self', in L. Martin, H. Gutman and P. Hutton (eds) *Technologies of the Self: a Seminar with Michel Foucault,* London: Tavistock.

___ (1990a) *The Care of the Self: the History of Sexuality Volume Three,* London: Penguin.

___ (1990b) *The Use of Pleasure: Volume Two of The History of Sexuality,* New York: Vintage Books.

Fox, N. (2001) 'Use of the Internet by medical voluntary groups in the UK', *Social Science and Medicine* 52: 155–6.

Fox, R. (1988) *Essays in Medical Sociology: Journeys into the Field,* New Brunswick, NJ: Transaction Books.

Freeman, J. (1994) 'I want to be happy too', *The Age* 5 June: 1.

Freidson, E. (1961) *Patients' Views of Medical Practice,* New York: Russell Sage Foundation.

___ (1970) *Profession of Medicine: a Study in the Sociology of Applied Knowledge,* New York: Dodd Mead.

Freud, S. (1985) 'Civilization and its discontents', in A. Dickson (ed.) *Civilization, Society and Religion: Group Psychology, Civilization and its Discontents and Other Works,* London: Pelican.

Freund, P. and Fisher, M. (1982) *The Civilized Body: Social Domination, Control and Health,* Philadelphia: Temple University Press.

Fries, J.F., Koop, C.E., Sokolov, J., Beadle, C.E. and Wright, D. (1998) 'Beyond health promotion: reducing need and demand for medical care', *Health Affairs* 17, 2: 70–84.

Fuchs, V. (1974) *Who Shall Live? Health, Economics and Social Choice,* New York: Basic Books.

Fulder, S. (1988) *The Handbook of Complementary Medicine*, Sevenoaks: Coronet Books.

Furnham, A. (1994) 'The Barnum effect in medicine', *Complementary Therapies in Medicine* 2: 1–4.

___ (2000) 'How the public classify complementary medicine: a factor analytic study', *Complementary Therapies in Medicine* 8: 82–7.

Furnham, A. and Bhagrath, R. (1993) 'A comparison of health beliefs and behaviours of clients of orthodox and complementary medicine', *British Journal of Clinical Psychology* 32: 237–46.

Furnham, A. and Smith, C. (1988) 'Choosing alternative medicine: a comparison of the beliefs of patients visting a general practitioner and a homeopath', *Social Science and Medicine* 26: 685–9.

Gabe, J. (1995) 'Health, medicine and risk: the need for a sociological approach', in J. Gabe (ed.) *Medicine, Health and Risk: Sociological Approaches*, Oxford: Blackwell.

Gartner, A. (1985) 'A typology of women's self-help groups', *Social Policy* Winter: 25–30.

Gartner, A. and Riessman, F. (1977) *Self-Help in the Human Services*, San Francisco: Jossey Bass.

Gawain, S. (1982) *Creative Visualization*, New York: Bantam.

Gevitz, N. (1982) *The D.O.s: Osteopathic Medicine in America*, Baltimore: Johns Hopkins University Press.

___ (1988) 'Three perspectives on unorthodox medicine', in N. Gevitz (ed.) *Other Healers: Unorthodox Medicine in America*, Baltimore: Johns Hopkins University Press.

Gibbons, R. (1979) 'The evolution of chiropractic: medical and social protest in America', in S. Haldeman (ed.) *Modern Developments in the Principles and Practice of Chiropractic*, New York: Appleton-Century-Crofts.

Giddens, A. (1990) *The Consequences of Modernity*, Cambridge: Polity Press.

___ (1991) *Modernity and Self-Identity: Self and Society in the Late Modern Age*, Cambridge: Polity Press.

___ (1994a) *Beyond Left and Right: the Future of Radical Politics*, Cambridge: Polity Press.

___ (1994b) 'Living in a post-traditional society', in U. Beck, A. Giddens and S. Lash (eds) *Reflexive Modernization: Politics, Tradition and Aesthetics in the Modern Social Order*, Cambridge: Polity Press.

Glassner, B. (1989) 'Fitness and the postmodern self', *Journal of Health and Social Behavior* 30: 180–94.

Goffman, E. (1969) *The Presentation of Self in Everyday Life*, Harmondsworth: Penguin.

Goodheart, L. and Curry, R. (1992) 'A confusion of voices: the crisis of individualism in twentieth-century America', in R. Curry and L. Goodheart (eds) *American Chameleon: Individualism in Trans-National Context*, Kent, OH: Kent State University Press.

Great Smokies Diagnostic Laboratory (2002) *Introducing breakthrough genetic assessment for customized intervention*. Great Smokies Diagnostic Laboratory. Online Available HTTP *http://www.genovations.com/overview.html* (23 January 2003).

Green, L., Kreuter, M.W., Deeds, S.G. and Partridge, K.B. (1980) *Health Education Planning: a Diagnostic Approach*, Palo Alto, CA: Mayfield.

Habermas, J. (1981) 'New social movements', *Telos* 49: 33–7.

___ (1987) *The Theory of Communicative Action: the Critique of Fundamentalist Reason Volume 2*, Cambridge: Polity Press.

Haigh, G. (1995) 'Butt out: tobacco industry strikes back', *The Australian* 19 May: 29.

Halmos, P. (1970) *The Personal Service Society*, London: Constable.

Hannay, D.R. (1980) 'The "iceberg" of illness and "trivial" consultations', *Journal of the Royal College of General Practitioners* 30: 551–9.

Hardey, M. (1999) 'Doctor in the house: the Internet as a source of lay health knowledge and the challenge to expertise', *Sociology of Health and Illness* 21, 6: 820–35.

Haug, M. and Lavin, B. (1981) *Consumerism in Medicine: Challenging Physician Authority*, Beverly Hills: Sage.

Hay, L. (1988) *You Can Heal Your Life*, Concord, Australia: Specialist Publications.

Health Issues Centre (1991) *Self-Help Groups and the Role They Play in the Community*, Melbourne: Health Issues Centre.

Heelas, P. (1982) 'Californian self religions and socializing the subject', in E. Barker (ed.) *New Religious Movements: a Perspective for Understanding Society*, New York: Edwin Mellen Press.

―― (1992) 'The sacralization of the self and New Age capitalism', in N. Abercrombie and A. Warde (eds) *Social Change in Contemporary Britain*, Cambridge: Polity Press.

―― (1996) *The New Age Movement: the Celebration of the Self and the Sacralization of Modernity*, Oxford and Cambridge, MA: Blackwell.

Hildreth, A. (1942) *The Lengthening Shadow of Andrew Taylor Still*, Kirksville, MO: Journal Printing.

Himmel, W., Schulte, M. and Kochen, M. (1993) 'Complementary medicine: are patients' expectations being met by their general practitioners?', *British Journal of General Practice* 43, 371: 232–5.

Hitch, P.J., Fielding, R.G. and Llewelyn, S.P. (1994) 'Effectiveness of self-help and support groups for cancer patients: a review', *Psychology and Health* 9, 6: 437–48.

Hochschild, A.R. (1983) *The Managed Heart: the Commercialization of Human Feeling*, Berkeley: University of California Press.

―― (1994) 'The commercial spirit of intimate life and the abduction of feminism: signs from women's advice books', *Theory, Culture and Society* 11: 1–24.

Holden, C. (1978) 'Holistic health concepts gaining momentum', *Science* 200: 1029.

Homola, S. (1963) *Bonesetting, Chiropractic and Cultism*, Panama City, FL: Critique Books.

Hooper, J. and Teresi, D. (1990) *Would the Buddha Wear a Walkman? A Catalogue of Revolutionary Tools for Higher Consciousness*, New York: Simon and Schuster.

Horkheimer, M. (1972) *Critical Theory*, New York: Seabury Press.

Horney, K. (1937) *The Neurotic Personality of Our Time*, New York: Norton.

Hubbard, B.M. (1991) 'The evolutionary journey', in W. Bloom (ed.) *The New Age: An Anthology of Essential Writings*, London: Rider.

Hughes, M. (1994) 'The risks of lifestyle and the diseases of civilization', *Annual Review of Health Social Sciences* 4: 57–78.

Illich, I. (1976) *Medical Nemesis: the Expropriation of Health*, Harmondsworth: Penguin.

―― (1990) *Health as one's own responsibility: No, thank you.* Olympia, Washington: Evergreen, State College. Online Available HTTP*http://academic.evergreen.edu/curricular/hhd2000/Rita/RESPONSIBIL.htm*(22 January 2003).

―― (1992) 'Twelve years after *Medical Nemesis*: a plea for body history' *In the Mirror of the Past: Lectures and Addresses, 1978–1990*, New York: Marion Boyars.

Jackson, T. (1985) 'On the limitations of health promotion', *Community Health Studies* 9, 1: 1–9.

James, P. (1996) *Nation Formation: Towards a Theory of Abstract Community*, London: Sage.

James, R. (1988) 'High tech/high touch: the self-care group and the healing process', *Health Promotion Journal of Australia* 3, 3: 269–76.

James, W. (1982) *The Varieties of Religious Experience: a Study in Human Nature*, New York: Penguin.

Jameson, F. (1991) 'Postmodernism, or the cultural logic of late capitalism', in L. McCaffery (ed.)*Storming the Reality Studio: a Casebook of Cyperpunk and Postmodern Fiction*, Durham, NC and London: Duke University Press.

Jason, L.A., McMahon, S.D., Salina, D., Hedeker, D., Stockton, M., Dunson, K. and Kimball, P. (1995) 'Assessing a smoking cessation intervention involving groups, incentives, and self-help manuals', *Behavior Therapy* 26, 3: 393–408.

Johnston, J.R. and Ulyatt, C. (1991) *Health Scare: the Misuse of Science in Public Health Policy*, Perth, Australia: Australian Institute for Public Policy.

Josefson, D. (1998) 'Marketing of antipsychotic drugs attacked', *British Medical Journal* 316, 7132: 648.

Kaskutas, L.A. (1994) 'What do women get out of self-help? Their reasons for attending Women for Sobriety and Alcoholics Anonymous', *Journal of Substance Abuse Treatment* 11, 3: 185–95.

Kass, L.R. (1975) 'Regarding the end of medicine and the pursuit of health', *The Public Interest* 40, Summer: 11–42.

Katz, A. (1993) *Self-Help in America: a Social Movement Perspective*, New York: Twayne Publishers.

Kavolis, V. (1970) 'Post-modern man: psychological responses to social trends', *Social Problems* 17: 435–48.

Kearney, J. (1991) 'The role of self-help groups: challenging the system and complementing professionals', *Health Issues* 28: 29–31.

Kerouac, J. (1958) *The Dharma Bums*, New York: Viking Press.

Kickbusch, I. and Hatch, S. (1983) 'Introduction: a reorientation of health care?' in S. Hatch and I. Kickbusch (eds) *Self-Help and Health in Europe: New Approaches in Health Care*, Copenhagen: WHO Regional Office for Europe.

Kiernan, V. (1998) 'Study finds errors in medical information available on the Web', *The Chronicle of Higher Education* 12 June: A25.

Knowles, J. (1977a) 'Responsibility for health', *Science* 198: 1103.

___ (1977b) 'The responsibility of the individual', in J. Knowles (ed.) *Doing Better and Feeling Worse: Health in the United States*, New York: Norton.

Krieken, R.v. (1992) 'The poverty of social control: explaining power in the historical sociology of the welfare state', in M. Muetzelfeldt (ed.) *Society, State and Politics in Australia*, Leichhardt: Pluto Press.

Labonte, R. (1997a) 'Power and empowerment: building transformative relations from the inside out', in R. Labonte and E. Reid (eds) *Power, Participation and Partnerships for Health Promotion*, Carlton South: Victorian Health Promotion Foundation.

___ (1997b) 'A story/dialogue method for health promotion knowledge development and evaluation', in R. Labonte and E. Reid (eds) *Power, Participation and Partnerships for Health Promotion*, Carlton South: Victorian Health Promotion Foundation.

Laing, R.D. (1965) *The Divided Self: An Existential Study in Sanity and Madness*, Harmondsworth: Penguin.

Lalonde, M. (1974) *A New Perspective on the Health of Canadians*, Ottawa: Department of National Health and Welfare.

Lasch, C. (1980) *The Culture of Narcissism: American Life in an Age of Diminishing Expectations*, London: Sphere Books.

___ (1984) *The Minimal Self: Psychic Survival in Troubled Times*, New York: Norton.

Last, J.M. (1963) 'The iceberg: completing the clinical picture in general practice', *Lancet* 2: 28.

Lears, J. (1989) 'American advertising and the reconstruction of the body, 1880–1930', in K. Grover (ed.) *Fitness in American Culture: Images of Health, Sport and the Body, 1830–1940*, Amherst and New York: University of Massachussets Press and the Margaret Woodbury Strong Museum.

Leichter, H. (1991) *Free to be Foolish: Politics and Health Promotion in the United States and Great Britain*, Princeton, NJ: Princeton University Press.

Leifer, R. (1969) *In the Name of Mental Health*, New York: Science House.

Levin, A. (1975) *Talk Back to Your Doctor*, New York: Doubleday.

Levin, L., Katz, A. and Holst, E. (1979) *Self-Care: Lay Initiatives in Health, Second Edition*, New York: Prodist.

Levine, M. (1988) 'How self-help works', *Social Policy* 19, 1: 39–43.

Levine, M. and Perkins, D.V. (1987) *Principles of Community Psychology*, New York: Oxford University Press.

Lidskog, R. (1996) 'In science we trust? On the relation between scientific knowledge, risk consciousness and public trust', *Acta Sociologica* 39, 1: 31–56.

Lillard, L. and Waite, L. (1995) ''Til death do us part: marital disruption and mortality', *American Journal of Sociology* 100, 5: 1131–56.

Linn, L. and Lewis, C. (1977) 'Attitudes toward self-care among practicing physicians', *Medical Care* 17: 183–90.

Lippman, A. (1999) 'Choice as a risk to women's health', *Health, Risk and Society* 1, 3: 281–91.

Lloyd, P., Lupton, D., Wiesner, D. and Hasleton, S. (1993) 'Choosing alternative therapy: an exploratory study of sociodemographic characteristics and motives of patients resident in Sydney', *Australian Journal of Public Health* 17, 2: 135–44.

Lowther, D. (1997) 'Collective of self-help groups', *Health Issues* 51: 6.

Lupton, D. (1994) *Health Promotion, Moral Regulation and the Care of the Self*, paper presented at the Annual Conference of the Australian Sociological Association, Deakin University, Australia.

—— (1995) *The Imperative of Health: Public Health and the Regulated Body*, London: Sage.

Lyall, C. (1997) 'The Trade Practices Act and health providers: some implications for consumers', *Health Issues* 50: 17–20.

McClung, H.J., Murray, R. and Heitlinger, L. (1998) 'The Internet as a source of current patient information', *Pediatrics* 101, 6: e2.

McDonald, K. (1993) 'On work', *Arena Journal*, 2: 33–42.

McEwen, J., Martin, C. and Wilkins, N. (1983) *Participation in Health*, London: Croom Helm.

Machado, R. (1994) *Five things you can do to fight entropy now*. Transtopia. Online Available HTTP *http://meltingpot.fortunecity.com/kuwait/557/5things.html* (27 January 2003).

McKeown, T. (1976) *The Modern Rise of Population*, London: Edward Arnold.

—— (1979) *The Role of Medicine: Dream, Mirage, or Nemesis?*, Oxford: Blackwell.

McKeown, T. and Lowe, C.R. (1974) *An Introduction to Social Medicine, Second Edition*, Oxford: Blackwell.

McKimmie, M. (1995) 'Rothmans comes out fighting', *West Australian* (Perth) 16 May: 1–2.

MacLennan, A.H., Wilson, D.H. and Taylor, A.W. (1996) 'Prevalence and cost of alternative medicine in Australia', *Lancet* 347: 569–72.

Maddocks, I. (1985) 'Alternative medicine', *Medical Journal of Australia* 142: 547–51.

Marin, P. (1975) 'The new narcissism', *Harper's* 14 October: 45–56.

Marks, R. (1994) 'Skin cancer control in Australia: have we made any difference?', *Australian Journal of Public Health* 18, 2: 127–8.

Martin, L., Gutman, H. and Hutton, P. (eds) (1988) *Technologies of the Self: a Seminar with Michel Foucault*, London: Tavistock.

Marx, K. (1976) *Capital*, Harmondsworth: Penguin.

Mauss, M. (1973) 'Techniques of the body', *Economy and Society* 2, 1: 70–88.

___ (1979a) 'Biographical list of body techniques', in *Sociology and Psychology: Essays*, London and Boston: Routledge and Kegan Paul.

___ (1979b) 'The notion of body techniques', in *Sociology and Psychology: Essays*, London and Boston: Routledge and Kegan Paul.

Melucci, A. (1994) 'A strange kind of newness: what's new in New Social Movements?' in H. Johnston, E. Laraña and J. Gusfield (eds) *New Social Movements: From Ideology to Identity*, Philadelphia: Temple University Press.

___ (1996) *The Playing Self: Person and Meaning in the Planetary Society*, Cambridge: Cambridge University Press.

Milligan, R., Beilin, L.J., Dunbar, D.L., Spencer, M.J., Balde, E. and Gracey, M.P. (1998) 'Influence of gender and socio-economic status on dietary patterns and nutrient intakes in 18-year-old Australians', *Australian and New Zealand Journal of Public Health* 22, 4: 485–93.

Mishler, E. (1981) 'The social construction of illness', in E. Mishler (ed.) *Social Contexts of Health, Illness and Patient Care*, London: Cambridge University Press.

Mooney, G. (1995) 'Efficiency in health care: just health gains?' *Australian Journal of Public Health* 19, 4: 330–5.

Moorhouse, G. (1969) 'Psychiatrist of liberation', in H. Thomas (ed.) *The Permissive Society: the Guardian Inquiry*, London: Guardian Newspapers.

More, M. (1994) 'On Becoming Posthuman', *Free Inquiry* Fall. Online Available HTTP *http://www.maxmore.com/becoming.htm*

___ (1997) *Technological self-transformation: expanding personal extropy*. Online Available HTTP *http://www.primenet.com/~mazmore/selftrns.htm*

Murakami, H. (1999) *The Wind-up Bird Chronicle*, London: Harvill.

National Cancer Institute (1997) *Making Health Communications Work*, Bethesda, MD: National Cancer Institute.

National Health Strategy (1993) *Pathways to Better Health*, Canberra: National Health Strategy.

Newman, E. (2001) 'Medical publishing update: the Internet and the empowered patient impact the publisher/practitioner relationship', *Logos* 12, 1: 39–44.

Northcott, H. and Bachynsky, J. (1993) 'Concurrent utilization of chiropractic, prescription medicines, nonprescription medicines and alternative health care', *Social Science and Medicine* 37, 3: 431–5.

Nutbeam, D. (1998) *Health Promotion Glossary*, Geneva: World Health Organization.

Okun, T. (1992) 'They should be our people', *Social Policy*, Fall–Winter: 44–8.

O'Neill, A. (1994) *Enemies Within and Without: Educating Chiropractors, Osteopaths and Traditional Acupuncturists*, Bundoora: La Trobe University Press.

Orem, D. (1991) *Nursing Concepts of Practice. Fourth Edition*, New York: McGraw Hill.

Packard, V. (1957) *The Hidden Persuaders*, London: Longman.

Parenti, M. (1986) *Inventing Reality: the Politics of the Mass Media*, New York: St Martin's Press.

Parsons, T. (1951) *The Social System*, New York: Free Press.

___ (1958) 'Definitions of health and illness in the light of American values and social structure', in E.G. Jaco (ed.) *Patients, Physicians and Illness*, Glencoe, IL: Free Press.

___ (1975) 'The sick role and the role of the physician reconsidered', *Milbank Quarterly* 53, 3: 257–78.

Paterson, J. (1996) *National Healthcare Reform: the Last Picture Show*, Melbourne: Victorian Department of Human Services.

Patton, G. (1997) 'Research leads the way to new approaches to smoking prevention and cessation strategies', *Health Promotion Matters* 1: 8.

Percival, T. (1973) 'Observations on the state of population in Manchester, 1789', in B. Benjamin (ed.) *Population and Disease in Early Industrial England*, London: Gregg International.

Petersen, A. (1996) 'Risk and the regulated self: the discourse of health promotion as politics of uncertainty', *Australian and New Zealand Journal of Sociology* 32, 1: 44–57.

Petersen, A. and Lupton, D. (1996) *The New Public Health: Health and Self in the Age of Risk*, St Leonards: Allen and Unwin.

Petrakis, P. (1988) 'Research report of the Surgeon General's workshop on self-help and public health', *Social Policy* 19, 1: 36–8.

Pilisuk, M. and Parks, S. (1986) *The Healing Web: Social Networks and Human Survival*, Hanover, NH: University Press of New England.

Pratkanis, A.R., Eskenazi, J. and Greenwald, A.G. (1994) 'What you expect is what you believe (but not necessarily what you get) – a test of the effectiveness of subliminal self-help audiotapes', *Basic and Applied Social Psychology* 15, 3: 251–76.

Pratt, L. (1973) 'The significance of the family in medication', *Journal of Comparative Family Studies* 4, 1: 13–31.

Read, J. (1995) 'Fight back, smokers told', *Adelaide Advertiser* 17 May: 21.

Rieff, P. (1966) *The Triumph of the Therapeutic: Uses of Faith After Freud*, New York: Harper and Row.

Riesman, D., with Denny, R. and Glazer, N. (1950) *The Lonely Crowd: a Study of the Changing American Character*, New Haven: Yale University Press.

Riessman, F. and Bay, T. (1992) 'The politics of self-help', *Social Policy*, Fall–Winter: 28–38.

Rissel, C. (1991) 'Using mass media for health promotion', *Health Promotion Journal of Australia* 1, 2: 64–5.

Ritchie, J. (1991) 'From health education to education for health in Australia: an historical perspective', *Health Promotion International* 6, 2: 157–63.

Roberts, R. (1994) 'Power and empowerment: New Age managers and the dialectics of modernity/ postmodernity', *Religion Today* 9, 9: 3–13.

Robinson, T.N. (1999) 'Reducing children's television viewing to prevent obesity: a randomized controlled trial', *Journal of the American Medical Association* 282, 6: 1561–7.

Roe, M. (1984) 'Science in the practice of medicine', *Perspectives in Biology and Medicine* 27, 3: 386–400.

Rogers, A., Hassell, K. and Nicolaas, G. (1999) *Demanding Patients? Analysing the Use of Primary Care*, Buckingham: Open University Press.

Rogers, R. and McMillin, C.S. (1989) *The Healing Bond: Treating Addiction in Groups*, New York: Norton.

Rose, N. (1990) *Governing the Soul: the Shaping of the Private Self*, London: Routledge.

―― (1992) 'Governing the enterprising self', in P. Heelas and P. Morris (eds) *The Values of the Enterprise Culture: the Moral Debate*, London: Routledge.

―― (1993) 'Government, authority and expertise in advanced liberalism', *Economy and Society* 22, 3: 283–99.

―― (1996) 'Authority and the genealogy of subjectivity', in P. Heelas, S. Lash and P. Morris (eds) *Detraditionalization: Critical Reflections on Authority and Identity*, Cambridge, USA and Oxford: Blackwell.

Rose, N. and Miller, P. (1992) 'Political power beyond the state: problematics of government', *British Journal of Sociology* 43, 2: 173–205.

Rosen, G. (1987) 'Self-help treatment books and the commercialization of psychotherapy', *American Psychologist* 42, 1: 46–51.

―― (1994) 'Self-help task forces revisited: a reply', *Professional Psychology: Research and Practice* 25, 2: 100–1.

Rosenberg, C. (1977) 'The therapeutic revolution: medicine, meaning and social change in the nineteenth century.' *Perspectives in Biology and Medicine* 20: 485–506.

Rosenstock, I. (1990) 'Personal responsibility and public policy in health promotion', in S. Shumaker, E. Schron and J. Ockene (eds) *Handbook of Health Behavior Change*, New York: Springer.

Roszak, T. (1975) *Unfinished Animal: the Aquarian Frontier and the Evolution of Consciousness*, New York: Harper and Row.

Rottenberg, S. (1980) 'Self medication: the economic perspective', in *Self Medication: the New Era*, Washington, DC: The Proprietary Association.

Rowland, M. (1993) *Absolute Happiness*, Bondi Beach: Self Communications.

Ryan, J., Wentworth, W. and Chapman, G. (1994) 'Models of emotions in therapeutic self-help books', *Sociological Spectrum* 14, 3: 241–55.

Ryan, W. (1976) *Blaming the Victim, Second Edition*, New York: Vintage.

Salmon, J.W. (1984) 'Defining health and reorganising medicine', in J.W. Salmon (ed.) *Alternative Medicines: Popular and Policy Perspectives*, London: Tavistock.

Sawicky, M. (1992) 'What is NEWP? A guiding theory of the New Right', *Social Policy* 22, 3: 7–19.

Sawyer, M., Gannoni, A., Toogood, I., Antoniou, G. and Rice, M. (1994) 'The use of alternative therapies by children with cancer', *Medical Journal of Australia* 160: 320–2.

Schnert, K. (1975) *How to be Your Own Doctor (Sometimes)*, New York: Grosset and Dunlap.

Schwartz, H. and Biederman, I. (1987) 'Lay initiatives in the consumption of healthcare', in H. Schwartz (ed.) *Dominant Issues in Medical Sociology, Second Edition*, New York: Random House.

Seedhouse, D. (1997) *Health Promotion: Philosophy, Prejudice and Practice*, Chichester: John Wiley & Sons.

Sennett, R. (1974) *The Fall of Public Man*, Cambridge: Cambridge University Press.

Sethna, C. (1992) 'Accepting "total and complete responsibility": New Age neo-feminist violence against women', *Feminism and Psychology* 2, 1: 113–19.

Shapiro, E. (1983) 'The physician visit patterns of chiropractic users: health-seeking behavior of the elderly in Manitoba, Canada', *American Journal of Public Health* 73, 5: 553–7.

Sharp, G. (1985) 'Constitutive abstraction and social practice', *Arena*, 70: 48–82.

Sheehan, M. (1984) 'Attitudinal determinants of use of non-medical healers', in S. Camp-
    bell, J. Dillon and J. Jamison (eds) *Developments and Needs in Education and Social Science
    Research of Chiropractic*, Armidale: University of New England.
Shilling, C. (1993) *The Body and Social Theory*, London: Sage.
Siahpush, M. (1999) 'Postmodern attitudes about health: a population-based exploratory
    study', *Complementary Therapies in Medicine* 7: 164–9.
Silverman, D. (1987) *Communication and Medical Practice: Social Relations in the Clinic*, London:
    Sage.
Slater, P. (1976) *The Pursuit of Loneliness: American Culture at the Breaking Point*, Boston: Beacon
    Press.
Sloan, T. (1987) *Deciding: Self-Deception in Life Choices*, New York and London: Methuen.
Söderhamn, O. (2000) 'Self-care activity as a structure: a phenomenological approach',
    Scandinavian Journal of Occupational Therapy 7: 183–9.
Spiegel, D. (1989) 'Effect of psychosocial treatment on survival of patients with metastatic
    breast cancer', *Lancet* 2: 888–91.
Stanway, A. (1980) *Alternative Medicine: a Guide to Natural Therapies*, London: MacDonald
    and Jane's.
Starhawk (1979) *The Spiral Dance: a Rebirth of the Ancient Religion of the Great Goddess*, San
    Francisco: Harper and Row.
___ (1990) *Truth or Dare: Encounters with Power, Authority and Mystery*, San Francisco: Harper.
Stewart, M. (1990a) 'Expanding theoretical conceptualizations of self-help groups', *Social
    Science and Medicine* 31, 9: 1057–66.
___ (1990b) 'Professional interface with mutual aid self-help groups: a review', *Social
    Science and Medicine* 31, 10: 1143–58.
Still, A.T. (1899) *Philosophy of Osteopathy*, Kirksville, MO: published by the author
    (Academy of Applied Osteopathy facsimile edition).
Stokols, D. (1996) 'Translating social ecological theory into guidelines for community
    health promotion', *American Journal of Health Promotion* 10: 282–98.
___ (2000) 'The social ecological paradigm of wellness promotion', in M. Schneider
    Jamner and D. Stokols (eds) *Promoting Human Wellness: New Frontiers for Research, Practice,
    and Policy*, Berkeley and Los Angeles: University of California Press.
Strohman, R.C. (2000) 'Genetic determinism as a failing paradigm in biology and
    medicine: implications for health and wellness', in M. Schneider Jamner and D.
    Stokols (eds) *Promoting Human Wellness: New Frontiers for Research, Practice, and Policy*,
    Berkeley and Los Angeles: University of California Press.
Swan, N. (2002) *Anti-immunisation websites*. Australian Broadcasting Corporation. Online
    Available HTTP *http://www.abc.net.au/health/minutes/stories/s597729.htm* (24 January
    2003).
Swanwick, J. (1995) 'Lobbyist can't be fagged with passive stance', *Courier Mail* (Brisbane)
    19 May: 9.
Szasz, T. (1961) *The Myth of Mental Illness*, New York: Harper and Row.
Szasz, T. and Hollander, M. (1956) 'The basic models of the doctor–patient relationship',
    Archives in Internal Medicine, 97: 585–92.
Tamura, M. (1993) 'Healing case studies', *Psychic Reader (San Francisco)* December: 17.
Telford, R. (1993) *Take Care of Yourself: Your Personal Guide to Self-Care and Preventing Illness*,
    Sydney: Addison-Wesley.
Thomas, H. (ed.) (1969) *The Permissive Society: the Guardian Inquiry*, London, Guardian
    Newspapers.

Thompson, J. (1996) 'Tradition and self in a mediated world', in P. Heelas, S. Lash and P. Morris (eds) *Detraditionalization: Critical Reflections on Authority and Identity*, Cambridge, USA and Oxford: Blackwell.

Toffler, A. (1971) *Future Shock*, London: Pan Books.

Toumbourou, J. and Hamilton, M. (1994) 'Researching self-help drug treatment – collaboration and conflict in the age of harm reduction', *Addiction* 89, 2: 151–6.

Trojan, A. (1989) 'Benefits of self-help groups: a survey of 232 members from 65 disease-related groups', *Social Science and Medicine* 29, 2: 225–32.

Turem, J. and Born, C. (1983) 'Doing more with less', *Social Work* 28, 3: 206–10.

Turner, B. (1987) *Medical Power and Social Knowledge*, London: Sage.

___ (1991) 'The discourse of diet', in M. Featherstone, M. Hepworth and B. Turner (eds) *The Body: Social Process and Cultural Theory*, London: Sage.

___ (1994) 'Theoretical developments in the sociology of the body', *Australian Cultural History*, 13: 13–30.

Twaddle, A. (1979) *Sickness Behavior and the Sick Role*, Boston: Schenkman.

___ (1981) 'Sickness and the sickness career: some implications', in L. Eisenberg and A. Kleinman (eds) *The Relevance of Social Science for Medicine*, Dordrecht: Reidel.

Uljar, M. and Hendron, M. (1990) 'A collective notion of self-help', *Community Quarterly* 18: 6–13.

United Kingdom Expenditure Committee (1977) *Preventive Medicine*, London: Her Majesty's Stationery Office.

United States Department of Health, Education and Welfare (1979) *Healthy People: the Surgeon General's Report on Health Promotion and Disease Prevention*, Washington, DC: Government Printing Office.

United States Department of Health and Human Services (1980) *Promoting Health/Preventing Disease: Objectives for the Nation*, Washington, DC: Government Printing Office.

University of Queensland (1985) *Report to the National Chiropractic Consultative Committee on a Review of Chiropractic Services*, Brisbane: University of Queensland/Uniquest.

Victorian Government Social Development Committee (1986) *Report of the Parliament of Victoria Social Development Committee Inquiry into Alternative Medicine and the Health Food Industry*, Melbourne: Victorian Government Social Development Committee.

Waitzkin, H. and Waterman, B. (1974) *The Exploitation of Illness in Capitalist Society*, Indianapolis: Bobbs-Merrill.

Watkin, D. (1978) 'Personal responsibility: key to effective and cost-effective health', *Family and Community Health* April: 1–7.

Weitz, M. (1982) *Health Shock*, Feltham: Hamlyn.

Wentworth, W. and Ryan, J. (1992) 'Balancing body, mind and culture: the place of emotion in social life', in D. Franks (ed.) *Social Perspectives on Emotion*, Greenwich, CT: JAI Press.

White, P. (1960) *Voss*, Harmondsworth: Penguin.

WHO (1946) *Constitution of the World Health Organization*, New York: World Health Organization.

___ (1983) *Health Education in Self-Care: Possibilities and Limitation*, Geneva: World Health Organization.

Whorton, J. (1982) *Crusaders for Fitness: the History of American Health Reformers*, Princeton, NJ: Princeton University Press.

___ (1988) 'Patient, heal thyself: popular health reform movements as unorthodox medicine', in N. Gevitz (ed.) *Other Healers: Unorthodox Medicine in America*, Baltimore: Johns Hopkins University Press.

Wilkinson, S. and Kitzinger, C. (2000) 'Thinking differently about thinking positive: a discourse approach to cancer patients' talk', *Social Science and Medicine* 50: 797–811.

Williamson, J. and Danaher, K. (1978) *Self-Care in Health*, London: Croom Helm.

Willis, E. (1989) *Medical Dominance*, Sydney: Allen and Unwin.

Wilson, N., Quigley, R. and Mansoor, O. (1999) 'Food ads on TV: a health hazard for children', *Australian and New Zealand Journal of Public Health* 23: 647–50.

Wolinski, K. (1993) 'Self-awareness, self-renewal, self-management: learning to deal effectively with stress', *Association of Operating Room Nurses Journal* 58, 4: 721–30.

Young, T.R. (1972) *New Sources of Self*, New York: Pergamon.

Ziguras, C. (1997a) 'Paying your respects to someone else's elders: the Western appropriation of Asian and indigenous religious discourses', *Aedon: the Melbourne University Literary Arts Review* 4, 1: 67–87.

___ (1997b) 'The technologization of the sacred: virtual reality and the New Age', in D. Holmes (ed.) *Virtual Politics: Identity and Community in Cyberspace*, London: Sage.

___ (1998) 'Masculinity and self-care', in T. Laws (ed.) *Promoting Men's Health*, Melbourne: Ausmed Publications.

Zola, I.K. (1966) 'Culture and symptoms: an analysis of patients presenting complaints', *American Sociological Review* 31, 5: 615–16.

___ (1972) 'Medicine as an institution of social control', *Sociological Review* 20, 4: 487–509.

___ (1973) 'Pathways to the doctor- from person to patient', *Social Science and Medicine* 7: 677–89.

Zolo, D. (1992) *Democracy and Complexity: a Realist Approach*, Cambridge: Polity Press.

Index